Please Return to
Diabetes Clinic
408-972-3497
or Mary Hallum
972-6879 (Diabetes)
Clinic

D0098697

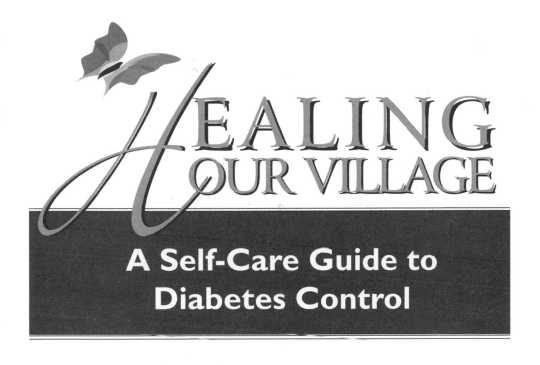

HEALING OUR VILLAGE

A Self-Care Guide to Diabetes Control

Lenore T. Coleman, Pharm.D., CDE
James R. Gavin III MD, PhD

HEALING OUR VILLAGE PUBLISHING
MARYLAND

Published, Distributed and Packed by: Healing Our Village Publishing

Editors:
Ikenna Myers, MD, MPH, CDE

Cover Design by: Mildred Baldwin

Book Layout and Design by: Tom Capossela

First Printing, January 2004
Second Printing, July 2007
Third Printing, July 2011
10987654321

ISBN 0-9746948-0-0

Healing Our Village Publishing
10104 Senate Drive #201
Lanham, MD 20706
www.healingourvillage.com
1-800-788-0941

About The Author Dr. Lenore T. Coleman 4
Acknowledgments Dr. Lenore T. Coleman 5
About The Author Dr. James R. Gavin III 7
Acknowledgments Dr. James R. Gavin III 8
Special Acknowledgments 9
Foreword by Dr. James R. Gavin III 11

Section 1 – DIABETES OVERVIEW 13
   Introduction 14
   About Diabetes 17
   Risk Factors for Diabetes 23
   Hyperglycemia 26
   Hypoglycemia 29
   Monitoring Blood Glucose and Blood Tests for Diabetes 33

Section 2 – DIABETES MANAGEMENT 43
   Diabetes and Nutrition 44
   Obesity and Exercise 66
   Type or Mode of Exercise 72
   Duration and Frequency of Exercise 74
   Management of Diabetes with Medication 79
   Oral Antidiabetic Medications 80
   Injectable Antidiabetic Medications 81
   Antidiabetic Medication Charts 98

Section 3 – HEALTH LITERACY 113
   Medication Adherence 115
   Tips on How to Talk with Your Health Care Provider 117

Section 4 - DIABETES COMPLICATIONS 125
   Complications of Diabetes 126
   High Blood Pressure 133
   Cholesterol and Heart Disease 144
   Understanding High Cholesterol and Its Treatment 147
   Smoking Cessation 160

Section 5 – OTHER COMMON CONDITIONS 167
   Types of Skin Conditions 168
   Taking Care of Your Feet 169
   Dental Care 172
   Erectile Dysfunction 174
   Depression 177

Section 6 – DIABETES IN THE WEST INDIES 185

Section 7 – GENERAL DIABETES INFORMATION AND RESOURCES 193

About the Author

Dr. Lenore T. Coleman, Pharm.D., CDE, FASHP

Lenore T. Coleman received her Doctorate of Pharmacy from the University of California, San Francisco. She completed an ASHP approved residency in Ambulatory Care at the USC School of Pharmacy.

Dr. Coleman has been a practicing pharmacist for 32 years. She has worked as a clinical pharmacist in the acute care, ambulatory care, long-term care, and community pharmacy setting. Within each of those practice settings, Dr. Coleman has focused on the care and management of people with diabetes and cardiovascular disease.

Dr. Coleman holds the title of Associate Professor, Xavier College of Pharmacy, Research Fellow, Center of Excellence, Howard University and A Certified Diabetic Educator of 15 years, Dr. Coleman provides education and drug therapy management to people with diabetes nationwide. She is co-owner of Total Diabetes Care and Medical Supplies and ADA Certified Diabetes Education Center, in the Greater Los Angeles Area.

In March 1996, Dr. Coleman became a Fellow of the American Society of Health System Pharmacists, which represents sustained excellence in a practice area for more than 10 years.

Dr. Coleman is currently the President and Founder of Healing Our Village of Maryland, Inc., **www.healingourvillage.com** a health communications company focused on eliminating health disparities through education and training of medically underserved patients and health care professionals.

Dr. Coleman is the Executive Director and CEO of Total Lifestyle Change, Inc. (TLC), a non-profit service organization that provides community outreach, advocacy and educational workshops throughout the United States, **www.tlc-global.org.** As part of TLC, Dr. Coleman has developed Project FAITH and Operation DETECT: A Cardiovascular Risk Reduction Program for Faith-Based Organizations. In 2004, she established Healing Our Village Publishing Company, in which *Healing Our Village: A Self-Care Guide to Diabetes Control* is the first of six anticipated easy-to-read health books.

Acknowledgements

I believe that we all have a purpose in life. Most of us wander through our lives trying to discover what that purpose is. Thankfully I recognize that my purpose in life is to reach as many people with chronic diseases, like diabetes, and give them the knowledge required to manage their condition successfully. There have been many influences in my life that have guided my path in this direction. The first and foremost is God—the Father, Son and Holy Ghost. Proverbs 3:5-6 tells us to "Trust in the Lord with all thine heart and lean not unto thine own understanding; in all your ways acknowledge Him, and He shall direct thy paths." To Him I give the glory for my career and success in life.

I would like to thank my co-author, Dr. James R. Gavin III for being both a gentleman and a scholar. Dr. Gavin is a leader in the field of diabetes management and prevention and he is committed to improving the health of the "VILLAGE." I truly appreciate your support and assistance in writing my first book.

My mother, Eleanor Ervestine Threadgill, was always there for me. For those who knew her they understood that she was "all business" and told you what she really thought. Thank you Mom for your generosity and for teaching me to always do my best.

I am very thankful for the people who mentored me early in my career, Horace Williams, James Wong, William C. Gong, Brad Williams, Mary Grear and Mary Anne Koda-Kimble. These exceptional pharmacists taught me to always strive for excellence in the field of pharmacy and to never be discouraged by the many barriers that we encounter everyday.

A special thanks to my close friends who have been there for me through "thick and thin." Deborah Williams, Robbie Butler, Anita Washington, Barbara Grant, Joy Childs, Zenobia Millet, Tobie Moree, Meredith Beal, Wayne Adams and Carl Betts. Thank you for helping me through the good and the bad times.

I am blessed to have two wonderful children, Ashley Corin and

Willie Akeem, who understand "the good of the many, outweigh the good of the few." They have always been there for me and support my need to help others and focus on my career. Thank you for your patience and unconditional love.

I would like to also thank my dear departed husband, Willie Otha Coleman. Through thirteen years of marriage, Willie taught me to always follow my dreams and that the needs of others should surpass your needs. Through this you demonstrate true love.

About the Author
Dr. James R. Gavin III MD, PhD

Dr. Gavin is a native of Mobile, Alabama, where he received his early education. He completed his B.S. degree at Livingstone College, a Ph.D. at Emory University and his M.D. at Duke University. His earliest involvement with diabetes was as a post-doctoral fellow at the NIH under Dr. Jesse Roth.

Upon completion of clinical training at Barnes Hospital, he held faculty and administrative positions at Washington University in St Louis, University of Oklahoma Health Sciences Center, and at the Howard Hughes Medical Institute in Chevy Chase, Maryland. He served as President and Professor of Medicine at Morehouse School of Medicine from 2002 to 2005, and prior to his current position as CEO and Chief Medical Officer of Healing Our Village of Maryland, Inc., he served as President and CEO of MicroIslet, Inc. in San Diego. He is Clinical Professor of Medicine at both Emory University School of Medicine, and Indiana University School of Medicine, where he also serves as National Program Director of the Harold Amos Medical Faculty Development Award of the Robert Wood Johnson Foundation.

He is a member of numerous honorific and professional societies, including the Institute of Medicine of the National Academies of Sciences. He is a past president of the American Diabetes Association, and chairman emeritus of the National Diabetes Education Program (NDEP). He is Chairman of the Board for the Partnership for a Healthier America, Inc. He has won numerous awards, including being named a Living Legend in Diabetes by the American Association of Diabetes Educators in 2009. He has authored more than 220 manuscripts, book chapters and scientific abstracts. He is married to Dr. Annie J. Gavin and is the father of three adult sons.

Acknowledgements

I would like to thank Dr. Lenore Coleman for her gifts of vision, creativity, and passionate commitment. Her boundless energy serves as fuel for my continued enthusiasm to continue this quest to reduce health disparities.

Simply saying thank you to my loving wife, Dr. Ann Gavin, falls way short of acknowledging the depth, duration, and impact of your unwavering love and support. To our sons Arthur (and his wife, Nicole), Rapheal, and Lamar, I extend thanks for their love and support and for the many times they have provided so much joy and laughter to this family and so much patience with me. My grand-daughter Racheal Anne has been a source of incomparable delight and I am especially pleased to acknowledge her inspiration and unconditional love, which has given me the encouragement I need to continue to pursue a world where diabetes will cease to be a source of dread and concern for our society and the human community.

I extend my deepest thanks to my many colleagues in NDEP, ADA, AACE, and AADE for their steadfast commitment to creating a better world for people affected by diabetes, and for the knowledge they have so unselfishly shared with me over the years. They have made me a better advocate for people with diabetes everywhere.

Finally, thank you Ms. Bonnie Claggett for the many years of excellent administrative and logistical assistance she has so expertly and selflessly provided.

Special Acknowledgements

As part of our third edition we are honored to have several of our professional colleagues contribute to the book. Currently, Healing Our Village is providing education and training in the Caribbean and Africa. We thought that the addition of a chapter on **Diabetes in the West Indies: Focus on Myths and Misconceptions** would highlight some of the similarities and differences in the way people with diabetes view their disease. We were delighted when Dr. Joel David Teelucksingh and Mrs. Zobida Ragbirsingh agreed to author this chapter.

In the technology area, Dr. David Horwitz, reviewed and contributed to our chapter on Blood Glucose Monitors. Fran Howell and Linda Mackowiak provided the chapter on insulin pumps.

My pharmacy colleague, Dr. Diane Ignacio, provided the updated information for all of the medication tables that appear in the book.

Detailed information on the contributors appears below. Both Dr. Gavin and I appreciate their input.

Dr. Joel David Teelucksingh is a Specialist in Internal Medicine with an interest in Endocrinology and Diabetes. He is a lifetime member of and scientific adviser to the Diabetes Association of Trinidad and Tobago. He graduated from the University of the West Indies and is a Member of the Royal College of Physicians in the United Kingdom. He has a passion for health education and voluntarily hosts television programmes and delivers public lectures on obesity and diabetes.

Mrs. Zobida Ragbirsingh is a retired registered nurse and midwife. She was also the District and County Health Visitor at the Ministry of Health. As a past North American region representative of IDF, past president of the Diabetes Association of Trinidad and Tobago and Diabetes Association of the Caribbean, she has been actively involved in diabetes education for decades. Recently, she completed her MSc in counselling.

David Horwitz, MD obtained his bachelor's degree at Harvard University, majoring in Chemistry and Physics, and has an M.D. and Ph.D. (in physiology) from the University of Chicago and an MBA from the Lake Forest Graduate School of Management. He is a Board-Certified internist and endocrinologist, and a Fellow of the American College of Physicians. He has published over 100 articles in scientific and clinical journals, primarily in the areas of diabetes and metabolism. Dr. Horwitz is presently Chief Medical Officer of the Johnson and Johnson Diabetes Institute.

Fran Howell, ND, APRN, CDE, CCRC earned a Bachelor of Science in Nursing from West Virginia Wesleyan College, Master of Science in Nursing from Marshall University and a Doctorate of Nursing from Case Western Reserve University. Ms. Howell is currently employed by LifeScan, Inc. as a Senior Manager, Clinical Affairs. Prior to joining LifeScan, Inc., she was employed by Animas Corporation as a Clinical Manager. Dr. Howell previously practiced as a Nurse Practitioner, Certified Diabetes Educator and Clinical Research Coordinator in two adult endocrinology practices.

Linda Mackowiak, MS RN CDE CCRA has worked as a family nurse practitioner, with a focus on the care of children with diabetes. She has worked in industry since 2000 in the field of continuous glucose monitoring, insulin pump therapy, and clinical research. She currently works at Animas Corporation as Senior Clinical Research Scientist in the Artificial Pancreas Program.

Diane Nadie Ignacio, Pharm. D. is a graduate from Howard University School of Pharmacy in 1998. She completed an Oncology/hematology Fellowship at the Howard University School of Pharmacy in 2009. A Registered Pharmacist in the State of Maryland she is currently a lecturer in Clinical Pharmacy and Therapeutics at The University of the West Indies, St Augustine Campus, Faculty of Medical Science, School of Pharmacy, Trinidad West Indies.

Forward

I vividly remember what a shock it was when I visited my beloved great grandmother in Selma, Alabama and found that she was bedridden, with one of her legs missing. I was just a young kid, but could recall earlier memories of her as a vibrant, kindly, and good-humored woman. Conversations among the adults were generally hushed when it came to any talk about the nature of her condition. The shock and puzzlement were intensified during the following summer, when the other leg was also missing, and she was no longer able to participate in conversations with us. One of the great joys of the visits to Selma had been the opportunity to talk with Mama Rennie—her stories were always fascinating. She died later that same year, and the only thing ever mentioned about why she died in those hushed conversations among the adults was "sugar."

As a kid I was puzzled about how something as good tasting as sugar could lead to the loss of a limb and the death of a loved one so full of life. I did not puzzle for long, because such questions did not appear to be encouraged and because it simply made no sense. Little did I know that I was now part of that village of people at risk and likely to be called upon to support someone affected. Years and years passed, and knowledge increased, and I became involved in diabetes and with such involvement came an understanding about "sugar." I came to know why we lost Mama Rennie—and so many others. These insights fueled my commitment to prevent such devastating impact of diabetes (sugar) on others. The urgency was heightened when it became increasingly apparent that there was a disproportionate impact of this disease in minority groups, including African Americans, and Latinos—major inhabitants of the village to which we refer in these writings.

I am very proud to join forces with my dynamic and committed colleague, Dr. Lenore T. Coleman, to produce this book. It is no longer necessary for persons with diabetes to suffer the outcomes experienced by my great grandmother. This serious disease can be treated and controlled, and its dreaded complications delayed or prevented. We simply did not know enough or have sufficient tools to help Mama Rennie in rural Selma back then. It did not matter that she was surrounded by a supportive and loving village. She herself was very much a take-charge sort of woman, but she did not know exactly what to take charge of or indeed just how. Well, we know now. We now know about better eating habits, exercise, and controlling blood pressure and cholesterol. We can communicate the essential information required to both prevent and control diabetes to the people with diabetes and to the VILLAGES that heal them.

This book represents our effort to speak directly to those who need to know the basics about diabetes, type 2 diabetes in particular, since this is by far the most common form in high-risk minorities. In addition, this is the form of diabetes most likely to be cared for by a primary health care provider instead of a diabetes specialist, and this is the form of diabetes where it is essential that the person affected assume front-line responsibility for self-care. The best outcomes are assured when such a person commits to self-care and is supported by a knowledgeable village—those who are committed to provide needed support.

This book is not intended to be an exhaustive treatise on the causes, consequences and interventions known to be important for people with diabetes. Rather, it addresses ground-level questions and essential every day information that enhances the ability for self-care. We have also included information about other helpful sources of information and toolkits to assist you in making important lifestyle changes for yourself and others in the village—those at risk. We are sure this will be a helpful guide to better control this growing disease in our village. We hope you agree.

James R. Gavin III MD, PhD.

Section 1
Diabetes Overview

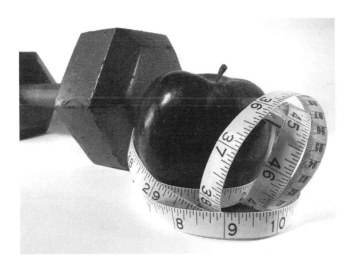

Introduction

Why did I get diabetes?

Why me? You may ask this question after you have been diagnosed with diabetes. You may feel that your life is over and your diabetes will control how you live. However, you are not alone. Diabetes is a very common problem for many people. In the U.S. 26 million people have diabetes. Approximately 19 million know they have it and 7 million are undiagnosed. In the minority populations, 3.7 million African Americans (14.7%) and 5.5 million Latinos (11.8%) have the diagnosis of diabetes. One in four African American women over the age 55 has diabetes. (Note: These numbers represent total prevalence of diabetes among people aged 20 years or older, United States, 2011.)

While we do not yet have a cure for this disease, diabetes is a treatable chronic illness. When properly educated and treated, you can live a long, productive life. This guide will provide information to help you control your diabetes.

Why should I learn about diabetes?

It is clear that control of this disease and prevention of complications requires day-to-day management. Patients must assume a major share of the responsibility for directing their care. Patients have demonstrated over and over that they are capable of taking charge of managing their diabetes when given the right kind of information, direction and support. Thus, it is absolutely essential that patients learn about management of diabetes.

How can I learn about diabetes?

Although diabetes is a complex disease, this self-care guide contains information that is easy to read and understand. Attending diabetes classes and support groups will help you learn "life saving information" and change the way you think about your diabetes. If you take control of your lifestyle, eating habits and medications you will be able to control your blood sugar and other risk factors and live a longer, healthier life.

This self-care guide has sections that discuss a wide range of topics related to your diabetes—sections about blood glucose (or blood sugar) monitoring, insulin use, use of diabetes medication, and foot care—just to name a few. It is important to discuss any questions you may have with your health care provider, diabetes educator, nurse, or pharmacist. While these health care professionals can help you control your diabetes, you are your PRIMARY CARE PROVIDER. You must assume the responsibility for your health and the health of your family.

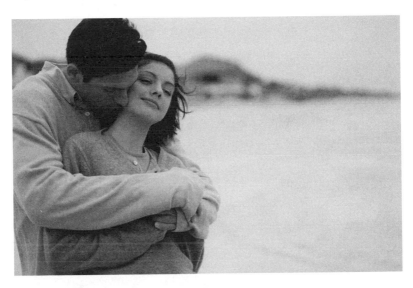

You are the most important person in the diabetes care team. All of the specialists in the world will not be able to get your blood sugar under control without your help.

All of the specialists listed in Figure 1 can help you manage your diabetes more effectively. Your family members and friends are also important in your care and management. Bring a family member with you to your medical appointment and diabetes classes so that they understand the many challenges that you face and can help and support you to make the lifestyle changes necessary to control your blood sugar.

Figure 1

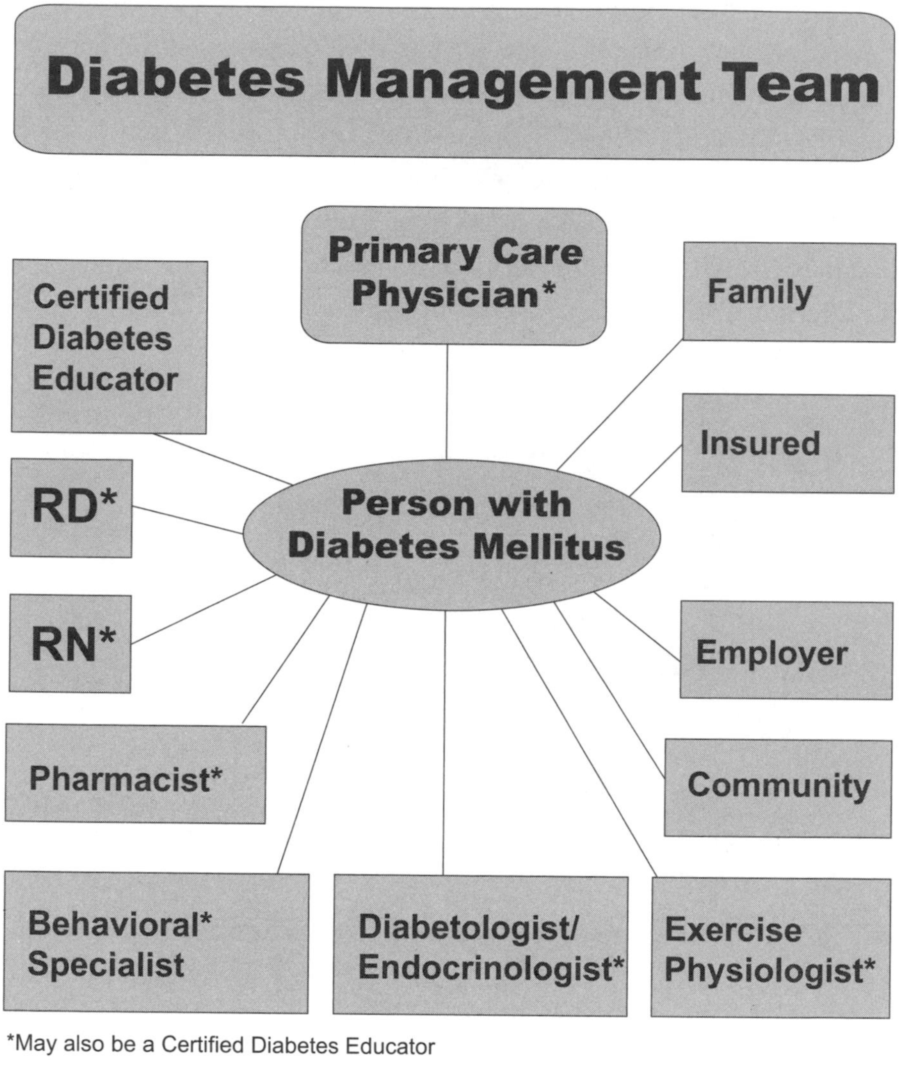

Diabetes Management Team

- Primary Care Physician*
- Certified Diabetes Educator
- Family
- RD*
- Insured
- Person with Diabetes Mellitus
- RN*
- Employer
- Pharmacist*
- Community
- Behavioral* Specialist
- Diabetologist/ Endocrinologist*
- Exercise Physiologist*

*May also be a Certified Diabetes Educator

About Diabetes

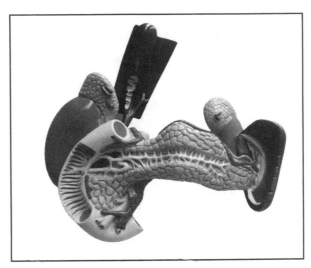

Model of a Pancreas

What is diabetes?

Diabetes is a disease that changes the way our bodies use food. People normally produce a protein hormone called insulin. Insulin is stored in your pancreas which is located behind the stomach. It helps the body to lower the amount of glucose, or sugar, in the blood, allows the body to use blood glucose for energy and helps store the glucose for future use. When your body is unable to make enough insulin or cannot use the insulin that it makes, the cells of the body cannot use the glucose for energy or fuel. People with diabetes may have little or no insulin at all. Sometimes their bodies have what should be enough insulin, but the body does not use it properly. People with diabetes have problems with other hormones in their body that are important for helping insulin to have its greatest effects to control blood sugar. All of these problems are targets for treatment in diabetes. Once you have been diagnosed with diabetes you must manage it for the rest of your life.

Everyone's blood glucose goes up and down every day in response to eating, exercise, stress, illness, etc. People with diabetes are different, in that their blood glucose is high and stays high if left untreated.

In people affected with diabetes, the high blood glucose levels may eventually damage the eyes, kidneys, small and large blood vessels, and nerves.

Diabetes is a progressive disease that actually begins in many patients as impaired fasting glucose (IFG) or impaired glucose tolerance (IGT). Impaired fasting glucose is diagnosed when the fasting blood glucose is between 100 mg/dL to 126 mg/dL. IGT is diagnosed when the blood glucose is 140 mg/dL to 199 mg/dL at the two-hour mark after liquid glucose is given to the patient. On March 27, 2002, the American Diabetes Association (ADA) released a "NEW" category called "Pre-Diabetes." Pre-Diabetes is a new word coined by the ADA and National Institute for Digestive, Diabetes and Kidney Disease (NIDDK) that combines IFG (blood sugars before meals blood greater than 100 mg/dL but less than 126 mg/dL) and IGT (after a glucose challenge) between 140 mg/dL and 199 mg/dL). People with "Pre-Diabetes" have a higher likelihood than others of developing diabetes. They also have a two-fold increased risk for heart disease.

Table 1. Classification of Diagnostic Categories

A1C _6.5%. The test should be performed in a laboratory using a method that is NGSP certified and standardized to the DCCT assay.*	or	FPG _126 mg/dl (7.0 mmol/l). Fasting is defined as no caloric intake for at least 8 h.*	or	2-h plasma glucose _200 mg/dl (11.1 mmol/l) during an OGTT. The test should be performed as described by the World Health Organization, using a glucose load containing the equivalent of 75 g anhydrous glucose dissolved in water.*	or	In a patient with classic symptoms of hyperglycemia or hyperglycemic crisis, a random plasma glucose _200 mg/dl (11.1 mmol/l)

*In the absence of unequivocal hyperglycemia, result should be confirmed by repeat testing.

The diagnosis of diabetes is made when your fasting blood sugar is greater than or equal to 126 mg/dL on two occasions or if your level is over 200 mg/dL after swallowing a standard solution of glucose in what is called a glucose tolerance test, administered by a health provider. Diabetes can also be diagnosed when a random (any time of day) blood sugar is over 200 mg/dL and classic symptoms of diabetes are present. The newest way to diagnose diabetes is when the A1C number is 6.5% or higher in many people (Table 1). For most people, diabetes is present without any symptoms for a period of 6.9 years.

Diabetes is a life-long illness that requires close control and watchfulness. You can avoid many serious medical problems by controlling your blood glucose (sugar). Taking care of yourself by keeping your blood glucose (sugar) as close to normal levels, along with regular visits to your health care provider, will help you have a full and active life with fewer complications.

Why should you be concerned about diabetes?

Diabetes is a serious, but treatable illness. Early detection and treatment are important in preventing many of the problems associated with this disease. There are signs to look for which may suggest you have diabetes. This guide will help you learn more about the signs of diabetes and determine if you or your family member may need to be tested.

What are the signs of diabetes?

There are many possible signs of diabetes. You may not have diabetes if you have only one of these signs. If the signs do not go away or you have more than one sign, you should see your health care provider as promptly as possible.

- Always thirsty and hungry.
- Going to the bathroom many times a day (passing of urine)
- Weight loss (when not trying to lose weight)
- Blurred vision (not seeing things clearly)
- Always feeling tired or feeling tired more often
- Infections that happen again and again

- Always feeling tired or feeling tired more often
- Tingling (pins and needles sensation) or numbness in the hands or feet
- Infections that happen again and again
- Sores on the legs or feet that do not heal
- Nausea and vomiting (Type 1 diabetes)
- Some people do not have any of the symptoms of diabetes so it is important to have your blood sugar checked once a year— especially if you have a family history of diabetes

What kind of diabetes do I have?

Type 1 and Type 2 are the two main kinds of diabetes. Type 1 diabetes usually occurs in children and young adults. People with Type 1 diabetes do not produce insulin and must take insulin for the rest of their lives. If you have Type 1 diabetes it is important to carefully plan your meals so that they match your insulin dosing.

In the past, Type 2 diabetes usually occurred in adults over the age of 40. We are now seeing Type 2 diabetes occurring at a much younger age—even in children and adolescents. People with Type 2 diabetes are treated in a number of different ways and may or may not have to take insulin. Being overweight may lead to Type 2 diabetes in people who are at risk for this disease. Since weight loss is one of the main goals of treatment, your health care provider will suggest that you exercise and carefully plan your meals. If weight control and meal planning do not work to control your diabetes, your health care provider may prescribe pills or insulin shots to control your blood glucose.

What if you have questions or concerns about your or your family member's diabetes?

If you or your family members have concerns about diabetes, it is very important for you to discuss these concerns with your health care provider. At that time, the health care provider may arrange for you or your family member to have some tests.

Checking the amount of glucose in the blood may help your health care provider find out how well the diabetes is being controlled.

If you suspect that your diabetes or your family member's diabetes is not being controlled, you should do the following:

- See a health care provider.
- Ask your health care provider questions about your specific treatment goals.
- Educate yourself on diabetes.
- Follow your health care provider's advice.
- Follow your diabetes treatment plan closely.

Test Your Knowledge
About Diabetes

1. The prevalence of diabetes in the United States has continued to increase over the years. According to the latest statistics from the American Diabetes Association there are currently:

    a) 13 million people in the United States with Diabetes
    b) 16 million people in the United States with Diabetes
    c) 18 million people in the United States with Diabetes
    d) 26 million people in the United States with Diabetes

2. Insulin is a protein hormone that is stored in the pancreas. It helps the body to:

    a) Lower the amount of glucose in the blood
    b) Use blood glucose for energy
    c) Store blood glucose as energy for future use
    d) Helps with storage of fat

    1) a,b,c   2) b,d   3) a,c   4) all of the above

3. People who have "Pre-Diabetes" have before meal blood sugars greater than or equal to 100 mg/dL and/or after meal blood sugars between 140 mg/dL and 199 mg/dL. People with "Pre-Diabetes".

    a) Are more likely to get low blood sugar reactions
    b) Are more likely to develop diabetes
    c) Will always experience symptoms of diabetes
    d) Have a two fold increase risk for heart disease

    1) a,b,c   2) b,d   3) a,c   4) none or the above

4. The diagnosis of diabetes is made when the blood sugar is 126 mg/dL or greater on at least two occasions.

    TRUE   FALSE

Risk Factors for Diabetes

Who gets diabetes?

It is difficult to predict who will get diabetes and who will not. Health care providers have studied people with this disease for many years. Because of these studies, health care providers have a good idea what may lead a person to have diabetes. Diabetes risk factors are what a health care provider looks for when considering whether or not a person will get diabetes. The more risk factors a person has, the greater the chance that the person will develop diabetes. Most people who develop diabetes have one or more of the following risk factors.

Table 2. Risk Factors for Type 1 and Type 2 Diabetes

RISK FACTORS FOR TYPE 1 DIABETES
▪ Race (People from Northern Europe and Italy are more likely to have Type 1 diabetes; people from Asian, Latin American and Native American countries are less likely to have Type 1 diabetes)
▪ Either parent (not step parents) with diabetes, or brothers or sisters (not step brothers or sisters) with diabetes; the greatest chance is if you have a twin with diabetes
▪ Nutrition (possible infant exposure to cow's milk)
▪ Virus exposure (Coxsackie B, cytomegalovirus, rubella, and mumps)
▪ Stressful events

RISK FACTORS FOR TYPE 2 DIABETES
▪ Either parents (not step parents) with diabetes, or brothers or sisters (not step brothers or sisters) with diabetes
▪ Being overweight (weight greater than 20% of ideal body weight)
▪ Physically Inactive
▪ Race (African Americans, Latino/Hispanics, Asians and Native Americans are more likely to have Type 2 diabetes)
▪ High blood pressure (>140/90 mmHg)
▪ Stress associated with injury or illness
▪ In women, a history of diabetes during pregnancy or delivery of babies over 9 pounds
▪ People with the Metabolic Syndrome (3 of 5 of these criteria) · Waist circumference > or equal to 40" men and 35" women · Triglycerides >150mg/dL or drug therapy for elevated triglycerides · HDL-C (Good Cholesterol) < 40 mg/dL for men and < 50 mg/dL for women or drug therapy for low HDL-C · Blood Pressure > or equal to 130 mmHg or 85 mmHg or on drug therapy for hypertension · Fasting Glucose > or equal to 100 mg/dL or on drug therapy for elevated glucose

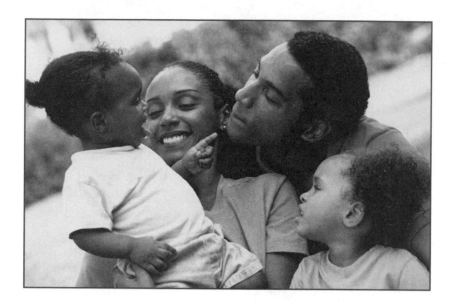

We know that diabetes runs in families. If you have diabetes, it is important to have all of your family members screened. By decreasing the risk factors, you can possibly delay the onset of the disease. Encourage everyone in your family to eat healthy foods and exercise regularly.

Test Your Knowledge
Risk Factors

1. The risk factors for Type 1 diabetes include:

   a) Race
   b) Possible exposure to cow's milk
   c) Virus infections
   d) Stress

   1) a,b,c
   2) a,c
   3) b,d
   4) all of the above

2. In Type 2 diabetes there are several risk factors that are not seen in Type 1 diabetes. These risk factors are:

   a) Family history
   b) Metabolic Syndrome
   c) Race
   d) Being overweight

   1) a,b,c
   2) a,c
   3) b,d
   4) all of the above

Hyperglycemia

What is high blood glucose?

High blood glucose (hyperglycemia) means that your blood glucose is higher than normal and is not coming down as expected. The symptoms of high blood glucose are the same symptoms that you had when you found out you had diabetes. These symptoms include the following:

- Frequent thirst or hunger
- Tired or sleepy
- Frequent trips to the bathroom (passing of urine, especially at night)
- Blurry vision
- Infections that come back again and again
- Slow healing sores or cuts
- Dry or itchy skin

When you have diabetes, eating more food than your meal plan calls for, or missing doses of medicine (oral diabetes pills or insulin) may cause high blood glucose. Getting sick, not exercising, or being stressed may also cause high blood glucose. High blood glucose levels and low blood glucose levels are both dangerous. In the long term, consistently high blood glucose levels will lead to the complications of diabetes, which directly impacts your quality of life. Low blood glucose levels, if untreated, can possibly lead to coma or death. It is important to keep glucose levels as close to normal as possible.

What can I do about high blood glucose?

The best way to treat high blood glucose is to first identify the cause. As a person with diabetes, if your glucose levels were in "control" and they become elevated, chances are, the cause is due to a change in your daily routine. You should follow your meal plan, get the proper exercise, take your medicine correctly and on time, and check your blood glucose more often. In addition, try to avoid stress at home and at work. If these things do not bring your blood glucose under control, call your health care provider for help. Your healthcare team may want to change your medication, change how much medication you are taking, or change how you take your medication.

It is important to note, in Type 2 diabetes, there is a progressive loss of the body's ability to make insulin over time, so there is a tendency for the disease to worsen with time. This means that the treatment must be adjusted periodically (increasing doses or combinations of medicines) to maintain glucose control. Many people with type 2 diabetes will eventually require some insulin as part of their treatment, which is a perfectly normal and expected stage in the natural history of diabetes.

Test Your Knowledge

Hyperglycemia

1. The common symptoms of high blood glucose (hyperglycemia) include:

   a) Frequent thirst and hunger
   b) Frequent urination
   c) Slow healing of cuts or sores
   d) Palpitations (heart beating fast)

   1) a,b,c
   2) a,c
   3) b,d
   4) none of the above

2. Your blood sugar can increase if you:

   a) Miss your diabetes medications
   b) Get sick with the flu or an infection
   c) Eat a larger meal than normal
   d) Exercise

   1) a,b,c
   2) a,c
   3) b,d
   4) none of the above

3. Diabetes is a progressive disease, which causes the blood sugar to increase over time.

   TRUE   FALSE

Hypoglycemia

What is hypoglycemia?

Low blood glucose (hypoglycemia) is a term to describe a blood glucose reading of less than 70 mg/dL. For most people with diabetes, low blood glucose also brings about some very unpleasant physical changes. If you experience a low blood sugar (glucose) reaction, you may experience the following symptoms:

- Shaky feeling
- Sweaty
- Headache
- Hungry
- Tired

- Confused or angry feelings
- Loss of consciousness ('pass out')
- Faster heartbeat
- Numbness or tingling in lips or mouth

Taking too much anti-diabetes medicine (insulin or oral diabetes medication) or getting too much exercise at the wrong times may cause low blood glucose. Skipping a meal or not eating enough or not eating meals at the planned time may also cause low blood glucose (especially if you are treated with medicines). If you feel any of these symptoms, do a blood glucose test to double-check. You should consider wearing a MedicAlert™ bracelet or necklace that states you have diabetes. There are also identification (ID) cards that you can carry in your wallet that provide similar information.

What do I do about low blood glucose?

If you experience any of these symptoms and sense that your blood glucose may be low, test it by using the blood glucose monitor. If for some reason your monitor is not available, you should eat or drink something containing a quick burst of sugar. There are several products available at your pharmacy that can provide this needed sugar. It is amazing to see that a little food or drink can actually help bring your blood glucose back to normal.

Your health care provider might recommend that you follow the 15:15 rule for treating hypoglycemia. Using this approach, you should ingest 15 grams of carbohydrate (CHO), wait 15 minutes and re-check your blood sugar. Eating 15 grams of CHO should cause your blood sugar to rise by 30-45 mg/dL. If blood sugar levels do not rise or if symptoms of hypoglycemia persist, another 15 grams of CHO can be consumed. An easy way to provide 15 grams of CHO is to eat or drink the following foods/beverages for treatment of your low blood glucose:

- 1/2 cup of orange juice or apple juice
- 1 cup of milk (skim)
- 6 hard candies (must have sugar)
- 1 small box of raisins
- 1/2 cup of soda (not diet soda)

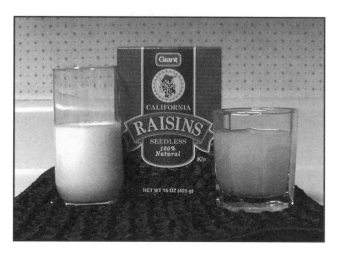

You can even eat several sugar cubes, a tablespoon of sugar or honey to help bring your blood glucose back up. You can also buy special glucose products at your pharmacy. These products are available in tablet or gel forms and are convenient to carry with you. These store-bought products work just as well as regular sugar to help bring your blood glucose back to normal. They also have a predetermined amount of sugar in the amount known to correct hypoglycemia in most people.

As noted in the 15:15 rule above, If you do not feel better in about 15 minutes, take additional food or drink containing sugar. If this second dose of sugar does not help, you should see your health care provider right away or go to an emergency room.

Sometimes blood glucose levels that are too low can cause you to pass out. It is important that your caregivers (family, friends and coworkers) not give you anything by mouth for your blood glucose if you have passed out. You may choke on it since you cannot swallow. In these cases, you should use an injection of a special protein hormone called glucagon. Your health care provider should give you a prescription for a glucagon kit, which you get at your pharmacy. If you take insulin, you should also have glucagon on hand. Since you will not be able to give the injection, someone in your family or a close friend (caregivers) needs to know how to give this shot to you. If you pass out, your support team should give you glucagon even if they are unsure if your blood glucose is low.

Test Your Knowledge
Hypoglycemia

1. Hypoglycemia is a term used to describe a blood sugar reading greater than 70 mg/dL

    TRUE   FALSE

2. The symptoms of hypoglycemia include:

    a) Headache, faster heartbeat, confusion
    b) Sweaty, shaky feeling, tired
    c) Numbness in the lips, blurred vision, loss of consciousness
    d) Palpitations (heart beating fast)

    1) a,b,c   2) b,d   3) a,c   4) all of the above

3. If you have diabetes it is important not to skip a meal and to eat meals at a planned time.
    TRUE   FALSE

4. The treatment of a low blood sugar reaction includes:

    a) ½ cup of apple juice
    b) 1 cup of skim milk
    c) 1 box of raisins
    d) 6 sugar free candies

    1) a,b,c   2) b,d   3) a,c   4) none of the above

5. If you pass out from low blood sugar your family or friends should administer glucagon instead of giving you something by mouth.

    TRUE   FALSE

Monitoring Blood Glucose and Blood Tests for Diabetes

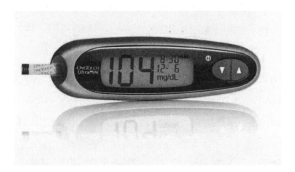

What is "control" and why should I control my diabetes?

"Control" means to keep your blood glucose (or sugar) level within the "target range" specified by your healthcare provider. Someone without diabetes usually has fasting blood glucose of between 60 and 99 (mg/dL). Although this "normal" range may not be routinely achieved or maintained, people with diabetes may come very close to this range with proper control. Keeping your blood glucose in goal range has been shown to help delay the complications of diabetes. These complications will be discussed in a later section.

What is a Hemoglobin A1C test and why do I need to have that test?

In addition to looking at your daily blood glucose readings, your health care provider may order a test that checks how well your blood glucose has been controlled over several months. This test is called a glycated hemoglobin or Hemoglobin A1c (A1C is the short name for this test). The A1C value is not affected by the time of day. The A1C value has been shown to predict your risk of developing many of the long-term complications of diabetes. Before the A1C test was available to your health care provider, they relied on the patient's record of blood glucose readings and other tests that gave them a "snapshot" of diabetes control. The A1C test gives your health care provider a better overall picture of how well your diabetes is being controlled over a long period of time and how closely you are following your treatment plan.

However, it cannot identify specific high or low glucose values, so is not a complete measure of how well you are achieving your glucose targets.

People without diabetes have an A1C of anywhere from 4% to 6% while people with uncontrolled diabetes may have an A1C of 8% to 18%. Various factors can change the results of the A1C test:

- Anemia (low blood volume) – decreases A1C values

- Short-term blood loss – decreases A1C values

- Use of vitamins C and E – decreases A1C values

This test requires no special direction for you to follow. You can eat before this test unlike some of the other blood glucose tests your health care provider orders. Do not be afraid to have this test done. You may have "good days" where your blood glucose is very well controlled. Along with those "good days," you may have some days when it is very hard to control your blood glucose. If the results from your A1C test are good, you should feel happy about how well you have been controlling your diabetes overall during the past 3-4 months.

What does the A1C value mean?

The A1C is measured in percent. The number represents your average blood sugar over 2-3 months. The following table gives you an idea of what your average blood sugar would be for each A1C percent value.

Table 3. Correlation of A1C with Average Glucose
Diabetes Care. December 30, 2010, vol. 34 Supplement 1 S11-S61

A1C (%)	Mean Plasma Glucose (eAG)	
	mg/dl	mmol/l
6	126	7.0
7	154	8.6
8	183	10.2
9	212	11.8
10	240	13.4
11	269	14.9
12	298	16.5

These estimates are based on ADAG data of _2,700 glucose measurements over 3 months per A1C measurement in 507 adults with type 1, type 2, and no diabetes. The correlation between A1C and average glucose was 0.92 (51). A calculator for converting A1C results into estimated average glucose (eAG), in either mg/dl or mmol/l, is available at http://professional.diabetes.org/eAG.

What is the target value for Blood Glucose Values and A1C

The following table shows some of the common ranges, goals, and treatment levels for blood glucose and A1C tests. It is important to note that this table contains numbers considered to be ideal goals for most people and is an example to look at, but may not apply to the goals set by you and your health care provider.

Table 4. Goals for Blood Glucose Values and A1C

TEST USED*	VALUE FOR PEOPLE WITHOUT DIABETES	GOAL FOR PEOPLE WITH DIABETES
Blood glucose Before meals (mg/dL)	Less than 115**	Between 70 and 130
Blood glucose At bedtime (mg/dL)	Less than 120	Between 110 and 150
A1C (%)	Less than 6	Less than 7

*Blood capillary plasma glucose measured in milligrams per deciliter (mg/dL)
(See page 36) and Hemoglobin A1C measured in percent (%).
**After an overnight fast, pre-beskfast values are usually below 100 in people
without diabetes.

There are many reasons for you to control your diabetes and get to your target goal for A1C. First, if you keep your blood sugar under "good control" (AS CLOSE TO NORMAL AS POSSIBLE), you can possibly prevent or even delay the long-term complications of diabetes and add years to your life.

Second, you will feel better when maintaining your blood glucose level at normal ranges. If your blood glucose gets too high or too low, you may feel tired, sick, and run-down. You need to pay close attention to your blood glucose range goals and A1C levels and stick to them with help from your health care provider, nurse, diabetes educator and pharmacist. Good control of your blood glucose can help you lead a healthy and productive life.

One of the most important components in the successful management of diabetes has been the patient's ability to self-monitor their blood sugars. In the past urine testing was used to assess blood sugar control. Urine tests for blood sugar were not good indicators of the blood sugar and their routine use was discontinued with the advent of blood glucose testing. Currently urine tests are only used for checking ketones in the urine especially during sick day management.

Blood glucose monitors and supplies are covered by most health insurance plans. It is important that you check with your insurance plan to make sure they cover the blood glucose test strips that you are using.

Why do I need to test my blood glucose daily?

Self-monitoring of blood glucose is one of the most important advances in diabetes management that has occurred in the last decade. All patients with diabetes should monitor their blood sugar. Monitoring of blood glucose is vital because it allows you to determine how well your body responds to the food that you eat and how well your medications are working. Blood glucose monitoring tells you if you need to increase your oral or injectable medications. Good control of your blood glucose levels will make you feel better along with preventing or delaying the long term complications of diabetes. Neglecting self-monitoring of blood glucose is like taking a trip across the country in a car without a gas gauge. Can you imagine? Would anyone do this? Monitoring your blood glucose helps to identify small upward trends in glucose levels before emergencies occur. As diabetes is a silent disease, most patients do not have symptoms of high blood sugar or they do not notice the symptoms. This is why it is so critical to check your blood sugar on a regular basis.

How often should I test my blood glucose?

How often you check your blood sugar depends on two things:

♦ *What type of diabetes you have (Type 1 or Type 2)and*

♦ *Are you at your target blood sugar?*

If you have achieved **"GOOD"** diabetes control (A1C< 7%), fasting blood sugars between 90-130mg/dL and you are not taking multiple injections of insulin, then you can monitor your blood sugar less frequently. Controlling your blood glucose helps avoid future problems such as eye and kidney damage. Talk with your health care provider or diabetes educator regarding how often and when to check your blood glucose.

In general, it is helpful to understand how your blood sugar changes during the day by getting a weekly "pattern." You can do this, for example, by testing before breakfast on Monday, 2 hours after breakfast on Tuesday, before lunch on Wednesday, 2 hours after lunch on Thursday, before your evening meal on Friday, 2 hours after that meal on Saturday, and at bedtime on Sunday. This will help your doctor decide on the best medication for you, and help you decide if the size of your meals is all right.

If you have Type 1 diabetes, you should check your blood glucose three or four times every day. Of course, if you adjust your fast-acting insulin with each dose, you need to test every time you are scheduled to take insulin.

It is important for you to alternate testing of your blood glucose before meals, two hours after meals and at bedtime. If you have Type 2 diabetes, you should generally check your blood glucose twice daily - less often if you are at glucose goals and stable, more often if you are not at goal and unstable.

If you check your blood glucose regularly it will help you achieve better control of your blood sugar. There are times when you may want to check your blood sugar more often. If you are pregnant, sick, or having problems with low blood sugar reactions then it is recommended that you check your blood sugar more frequently.

Lancets get dull, even after one use, and the duller they are the more they hurt, so you should remember to change the lancet in your lancing device. Your should never share your lancing device with another person because of the risk of spreading infection.

Which monitor should I use?

Most of the blood glucose monitors on the market provide fairly accurate results. Blood glucose monitors can become less accurate over time, so it is important to test the accuracy of your monitor occasionally (at least once a month) by using a control solution or check your blood sugar at the same time you have having your blood drawn at the laboratory. Keep in mind, the blood glucose levels drawn at the laboratory (called plasma glucose) is 15% lower than your reading from your finger tip (called your capillary glucose). However, most meters these days are now "fixed" or "calibrated" to match the laboratory reading. This may not be true if you have an old glucose meter.

Some monitors are easier to use than others, require a smaller drop of blood, and have fewer buttons, fewer steps to operate, do not require coding and take less time. You should work with your health care team, especially your diabetes educator to select the best monitor for you, but in general you should use a monitor that is easy to use, the numbers are easy to see, the meter does not require coding and has a memory function so that it records/stores your blood sugars. Your doctor may want you to use a meter that lets him download your results into his computer. And, of course, it should be a system where the strips are covered by your insurance plan.

How do I test my blood glucose?

It is a simple process to check your blood glucose. First, you need a drop of blood. If at all possible, wash your hands before testing, not only for cleanliness but to remove any sugar that might be there from foods you have touched--even things like fruit skins may have some sugar that can transfer to your fingers.

Prick your finger by using a lancing device. A lancet device is spring-loaded and fires the point of the lancet into your finger-tip with very little pain. Most lancing devices can be adjusted to the least depth required to give the size drop of blood you need. You may find that some lancing devices cause you less pain than others, so it is worth asking your diabetes educator about this. Gently squeeze your pricked finger to form a drop of blood.

Now you have your blood drop. You can check your blood glucose by using one of the many blood glucose monitors on the market. Most meters come with these steps clearly outlined to assure accurate use of these instruments.

Blood glucose meter testing

When you use your blood glucose meter, it tells you what the blood glucose reading is as a single number, not a range. Having a blood glucose monitor allows you to check your own blood glucose as often as you would like and determine the effects different activities or foods have on your diabetes during your daily life.

Your pharmacist or diabetes educator will also be able to help you prepare your blood glucose monitor for use and show you what supplies you will need monitor your blood sugar accurately.

Read the instruction booklet that comes with the blood glucose monitor very carefully. If you do a step wrong or miss a step, it could alter your blood glucose reading. Each machine has its own special kind of strips.

Follow the instructions for applying the drop of blood to the right blood glucose meter test strip. We recommend using a blood glucose monitor that has a memory function that stores your most recent blood glucose readings, along with a data management system that will give you a printout of your readings and provide a graph (picture) of your overall control.

Remember that glucose test strips are sensitive to light, heat, and moisture. Be sure to keep them in their original container so they retain their accuracy. Do not carry them loose in your pocket or purse.

Keeping track of your blood glucose

Your health care provider may ask you to keep a record of your blood glucose readings. You can track your daily blood glucose readings by using a Diabetes Self-Care Diary. This diary allows you to record the time, date, and results of each test. You can also record when you take your insulin and/or diabetic pills in your diary. It is important to bring this diary to your health care provider. This diary allows your health care provider to check your diabetes control and make changes to your treatment plan if needed. Being able to check your own blood glucose is one of the best skills you can use to control your diabetes.

When you visit your doctor, be sure to point out to him or her any glucose readings that concern you.

1. Check the expiration date on your strips before using them.

2. If you are using a meter that requires coding make sure the code is correct. Some studies have shown that an incorrect code can lead to blood sugar readings that are off by as much as 43%.

3. Follow the manufacturers' instructions on the proper use and care of your meter.

4. If using Alternative Test Site or forearm capillary remember that fingerstick readings do tend to be higher than forearm blood glucose readings after meals. Check with the health care provider or diabetes educator regarding the use of Alternative Site Testing.

5. It is important that you keep a daily record of your blood sugar readings. Every person with diabetes should have a logbook to record their testing results. We recommend the use of blood glucose monitors with data management systems that make tracking your results much easier since they have a memory. We recommend using a blood glucose monitor that stores at least 100 values in its memory.

Test Your Knowledge

Monitoring Blood Glucose

1. Controlling your blood glucose has been shown to delay the complications of diabetes.

   TRUE   FALSE

2. A normal blood glucose for people without diabetes is 60-99 mg/dL.

   TRUE   FALSE

3. Before having blood drawn for a hemoglobin A1C test, you need to:
   a) Fast overnight
   b) Not take your diabetes medicines that morning
   c) Avoid exercise for 24 hours
   d) None of the above

   1) a,b,c 2) b,d 3) a,c 4) all of the above 5) d only

4. An A1C of 7% represents average blood glucose of

   a) 120 mg/dL
   b) 154 mg/dL
   c) 170 mg/dL
   d) 270 mg/dL

5. The differences between the current blood glucose monitors include:

   a) Ease of use
   b) Different quantity of blood per test
   c) Fewer buttons and steps
   d) No coding and less testing time

   1) a,b,c 2) b,d 3) a,c 4) all of the above

Section 2
Diabetes Management

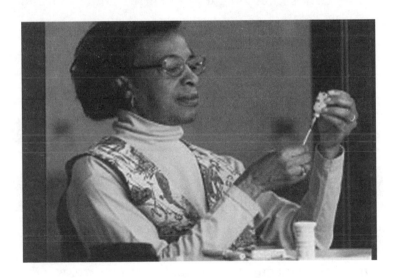

Diabetes and Nutrition
Introduction

One of the reasons for the dramatic increase in diabetes, especially in ethnic populations, is lifestyle. Poor eating habits and lack of exercise have contributed to significant obesity in many ethnic populations. Presently, over 60% of Americans are classified as overweight. Only 5% of all Americans who go on a "diet" and achieve their ideal body weight are able to keep it off after one year.

What is the role of food and nutrition in treating diabetes?

Food gives us the energy we need to live. Our body changes most of the food we eat into sugar called glucose that our cells need for energy. You can make a difference in your blood sugar control through your food choices. If you have diabetes it is important that you understand that you DO NOT need to eat or purchase special foods. Foods that are good for everyone are good for someone with diabetes.

What is Medical Nutrition Therapy (MNT)?

The control of blood glucose through diet is called Medical Nutrition Therapy (MNT). The goals of MNT include:

- Maintaining near-normal blood glucose levels by balancing your food intake with medications (either insulin or oral antidiabetic agents) and physical activity.
- Achieving optimal serum cholesterol levels.
- Maintaining adequate calorie intake to control weight gain and to achieve weight loss if necessary.
- Preventing and treating acute and long-term complications of diabetes.
- Improving your overall health.

Currently there are three popular food management programs that are used as part of MNT for people with diabetes—Carbohydrate (CHO) Counting, the Exchange System and the Plate Method.

Carbohydrate Counting is an easy concept to understand. The main nutrient in food that affects blood glucose levels is carbohydrates. Carbohydrates are composed of starches and sugars. They account for most of the glucose in the bloodstream. Only the amount of carbohydrate intake per meal is counted. Usually this is 45-60 grams per meal. Carbohydrates provide 4 calories of energy per gram. Carbohydrates should account for 45-65% of total daily caloric intake. The downside to using this method is that the focus is on carbohydrates. Fat and weight management are not initially addressed in CHO counting. In many ethnic populations, weight loss is essential to the prevention of future complications, so carbohydrate counting MAY NOT be the best method for some ethnic populations.

Table 5. Food Items High in Carbohydrate Content

Breads (rolls, pancakes, biscuits)	Desserts (cakes, pies and cookies)
Pasta (noodles and spaghetti)	Candy
Peas	Sodas, Punch, Kool-Aid
Potatoes	Ice Cream
Rice	Frozen Yogurt
Dry beans (pinto, kidney, lima and black eye peas)	Jams and Jellies
Lentils	Syrup
Milk	
Starchy vegetables	

What is the exchange system?

The exchange system provides patients a way of knowing which foods can be mixed and matched or substituted without changing the number of calories being taken in. The six exchanges lists help to make your meal plan work. Foods are grouped together on a list because they are alike. Every food on the list has about the same amount of carbohydrates, protein, fat and calories. In the amount given, all the choices on each list are equal. Any food on a list can be exchanged or traded for any other food on the same list. The six exchange groups are:

1. starch/bread
2. meat and meat substitutes
3. vegetables
4. fruit
5. milk
6. fat

Using the exchange lists and following your meal plan will provide you with a great variety of food choices and will control the distribution of calories, carbohydrates, protein and fat throughout the day, so that your food and your insulin will balance. The balance is what gives you "good" blood glucose control. Some of the common exchanges are shown in Table 9 and 10, which are located with other charts at the end of this section.

What is the Plate Method?

Many dieticians recommend the use of the plate method to help people with diabetes control their portion sizes while being able to chose the foods that you like. It's simple and effective for both managing diabetes and losing weight.

There are six simple steps to the plate method.

Step 1 — Take one of your smaller dinner plates and draw a line down the middle of the plate

Step 2 — Fill the largest section of the plate with non-starchy vegetables like spinach, carrots, lettuce, cabbage, green beans, tomatoes, cucumbers, turnips, etc.

Step 3 — In the other smaller section you put your meats like chicken, turkey, fish, or lean cuts of beef or pork

Step 4 — In the other smaller section you place your starchy foods like bread, rice, potatoes, pasta, sweet potatoes, peas, beans, etc.

Step 5 — Add an 8 oz glass of low fat or non-fat milk. If you don't drink milk you can try adding a container of light yogurt.

Step 6 — Add a piece of fruit for dessert.

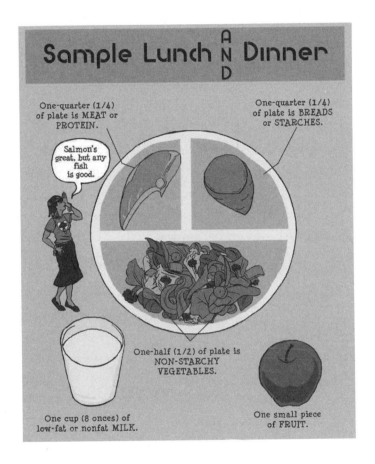

Protein

The body uses protein for growth, maintenance of muscle, skin and energy. Protein provides 4 calories per gram. Proteins should account for 15-20% of total caloric intake in patients with normal kidneys.

Table 6. Food Items High in Protein Content

• Meat	• Nuts
• Poultry	• Peanut Butter
• Fish	• Soy
• Cheese	• Dry beans and peas
• Starches	• Sour Cream
• Eggs	

Some vegetables have small amount of protein

Fats

Fats are a concentrated energy source. Fat provides 9 calories per gram, more than two times the calories you get from carbohydrates and proteins. There are different types of fat: monounsaturated, polyunsaturated, and saturated. Saturated fats have been linked to heart disease and have been found to increase your cholesterol levels. The "best" fats are monounsaturated and are found in olive oil, canola oil and peanut oil. Fats should consist of no more than 30% of daily caloric intake. Saturated fats should be limited to 7% of daily caloric intake.

Table 7. Food Items that Contain High Amounts of Saturated Fat

• Regular Milk	• Bacon
• Butter	• Red Meats
• Lard	• Regular Cheese
• Salad Dressings	• Sour cream

Trans Fat

Trans Fats are a type of unsaturated fat and can be either monounsaturated or polyunsaturated. However, while unsaturated fats (monounsaturated and polyunsaturated) are beneficial when consumed in moderation, saturated and trans fats are not. Trans fat occurs when the plant oils are hydrogenated. Hydrogenation changes the structure of the fat molecule and is used to change fat from a liquid form to a solid form. Trans fats can be found in small quantities in meat and dairy products.

Trans fats are listed on the label, making it easier to identify these foods. Unless there is at least 0.5 grams or more of trans fat in a food, the label can claim 0 grams. When reading the food label look for words like hydrogenated oil or partially hydrogenated oil. Eating *trans fat* can increase your risk for heart disease so you should avoid eating trans fat if possible.

Sources of trans fat include:

- Processed foods like snacks (crackers and chips) and baked goods (muffins, cookies and cakes) with hydrogenated oil or partially hydrogenated oil
- Stick margarines
- Shortening

Water

Drinking sufficient amounts of water every day is important to a well-balanced diet. Water is another nutrient that the body needs. It is recommended to drink eight glasses of water daily, unless otherwise indicated by your health care provider.

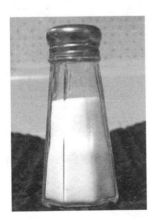

Salt (Sodium chloride)

Americans generally eat more salt than they need. Studies have shown that the average American eats 25 grams of sodium per day. Practically everything you eat contains salt. Make sure you read food labels carefully for the salt or sodium content. Avoid deli, processed and canned foods since they can be very high in sodium content. People with heart disease or high blood pressure should limit their sodium intake. The high sodium intake may contribute to high blood pressure in certain populations, especially African Americans. Most current national guidelines for diabetes and high blood pressure recommend limiting sodium intake to 2400 mg of sodium per day. Each meal should have no more than 800 mg of sodium, or no more than 400 mg of sodium per one food item. American Heart Association and American Diabetes Association recommend less than 2000 mg of sodium per day in patients with symptomatic heart failure.

Fiber

There are two types of fiber—insoluble and soluble. Soluble fiber helps to lower blood cholesterol levels, control blood sugar levels and may also help to control weight. Aim for a total fiber intake of 25-30 grams per day.

Table 8. List of Soluble and Insoluble Fiber Food Items

INSOLUBLE FIBER	SOLUBLE FIBER
• Bran cereals • Popcorn • Whole grain bread and cereal • Fresh fruit • Fresh vegetables	• Oat Bran • Oatmeal • Rice Bran • Barley • Dried beans and peas • Fresh fruit • Fresh vegetables

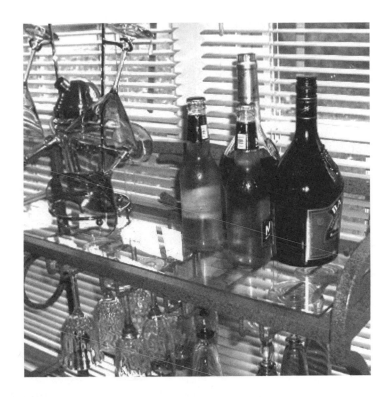

Alcohol use and diabetes

If you have questions about alcohol use you need to discuss this with your health care provider. In people with diabetes, alcohol:

- Provides calories and has no nutritional value. If approved by your health care provider it may be included in your meal plan but should be used sparingly to avoid weight gain.
- Can raise or lower blood sugar in some people with diabetes. When mixed with diabetes medications can cause unpleasant side effects such as nausea, flushing, sweating, or headache.
- Can dramatically lower the blood sugar when the person is on insulin.
- Should NOT be used if the person is taking Metformin.

The following guidelines should be followed if your health care provider says that alcohol CAN be included in your meal plan.

- Drink occasionally and only if your diabetes is "well controlled" (Note: Blood sugar goal should be 90–130 mg/dL).
- Use your blood glucose monitor frequently (2 times a day unless at goal).
- Have no more than the daily limit of one glass of alcohol for women and two glasses for men (1 glass = 4 oz. of wine, 12 oz. of beer, or 1.5 oz. of 80-proof spirits).
- Avoid sweet drinks, sweet wines, and liqueurs.
- Alcohol should not be substituted for food if you are taking insulin.

If you have diabetes, the following tips are important:

- You should eat small portions of a well-balanced, low-fat diet.
- Eat about the same amount of food at the same time each day.
- Try not to skip meals and incorporate small snacks into your meal plan. Skipping meals and snacks may lead to large swings in your blood sugar levels, especially if you use medication to control your blood sugar.
- The number of calories you need depends on your weight, height, age and activity level.
- Avoid "fad diets." Some high protein diets may actually cause you to have problems with your kidneys or may adversely affect your blood sugar.
- Try to maintain nutritional balance by including foods from all major groups, including carbohydrates, fats and proteins. Remeber, watch your portion sizes!

A healthy diet is important in controlling diabetes

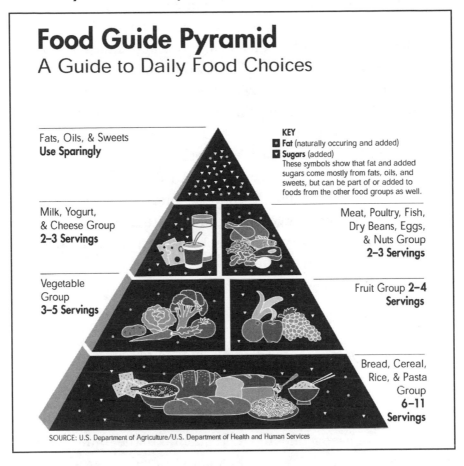

Food Pyramid from www.fda.gov

How do I get started eating a healthy diet and controlling my diabetes?

If you have Type 2 diabetes and are overweight (as most people are), the very first and most important change to make is to eat less at each meal and cut out in-between-meal eating. For more comprehensive assistance, the next step is to talk with a registered dietician to determine your daily nutritional needs and help you work out your own nutritional prescription. This plan will match the calories, carbohydrates, protein and fat you eat with your own physical activity level and with the insulin in your body. You and the dietitian will work out a specific meal plan just right for you. Your meal plan is a guide which shows the number of food choices you can eat at each meal and snack. As mentioned earlier the major reason for obesity in the U.S. stems from the fact that we eat **TOO MANY CALORIES** at each meal. Most women can achieve their ideal body weight by consuming 1200-1500 calories per day. Most men require 1800-2000 calories per day. You can eat more calories if you have a very active lifestyle and participate in moderate to vigorous exercise every day. Tables 11 and 12 at the end of this section provide you with a calorie chart and sample menus. Thinking ahead and planning your menu is very important. Preparation is the key to successfully achieving a lifestyle change. There are many books commercially available that provide a complete listing of foods and portion sizes for each food category. (i.e. starch, fruit, milk, vegetable, meat/ meat substitutes and fat).

What is the Glycemic Index?

This is a concept that is used by some nutritionists to control the blood sugar. Carbohydrates are absorbed into the bloodstream at different rates. The faster a carbohydrate is digested and absorbed into the bloodstream, the more rapidly the blood sugar rises. Rapid rises in blood sugar levels have been found to be detrimental to the lining of the blood vessels (endothelium) and may be linked to heart disease. The glycemic index is a measure or ranking of the effect of carbohydrate-containing foods on the postprandial (post meal) blood glucose response compared to a reference or test food. Glycemic indices range from less than 20% to over 120%. There are many factors that can affect the glycemic index of a food: the carbohydrate structure, fiber content, how the food is cooked or processed, storage, ingestion of other nutrients simultaneously, etc.

Foods that contain glucose or sucrose produce a large increase in blood glucose levels whereas foods that contain high amounts of soluble fiber decrease glucose absorption. When you eat foods with a high glycemic index your hunger may return more rapidly. Table 13 at the end of this section provides a partial list of the glycemic indices of some foods compared to one slice of white bread (= 100).

How do I read nutrition labels?

In order to maintain your calorie intake and not overeat, it is important to learn how to read the nutrition labels ("Nutrition Facts") that are found on the back or side of most foods. The nutrition label contains information on ingredients, serving size, servings per container, calories per serving, and detailed nutrient information. Total carbohydrate content is listed and broken down into sugars and dietary fiber. When reading the label for Carbohydrates or CHO:

- Check the ingredient list for sugar. When sugar is listed as one of the first three ingredients, most or all of the sugar in the product is added. If sugar is not listed in the ingredient list, then the sugar occurs naturally in the food.
- Sugar can be listed as: sucrose, maltose, fructose, lactose, glucose, dextrose, levulose, corn syrup, honey, brown sugar, cane sugar or molasses.
- Check the labels for sugar alcohol (sorbitol, mannitol, xylitol, maltitol, starch hydrolysate).
  - Products using sugar alcohol are often advertised as "No Added Sugar."
  - Sugar alcohol contains the same calories as sugar; however, it has a slower effect on the blood sugar.
  - Use only small amounts of these products and count the carbohydrates as part of your daily food allowance.
  - If you are having wide swings in your blood sugar then you should consider decreasing your carbohydrate intake and adding more fiber to your diet.
  - Check the label for total fat, saturated and trans fat. You should avoid foods that have more than 30% fat. You should avoid trans fats completely.

Nutrition Facts

Serving Size 2/3 cup (55g)
Servings Per Container 9

Amount per Serving	Cereal	Cereal with ½ cup Skim Milk
Calories	220	260
Calories from Fat	25	25
	%Daily Value**	
Total Fat 2.5g*	4%	4%
Saturated Fat	5%	5%
Cholesterol 0mg	0%	0%
Sodium 130mg	5%	7%
Potassium 40mg	1%	7%
Total Carbohydrate 46g	15%	17%
Dietary Fiber 4g	12%	12%
Sugar 16g		
Protein 4g		

DESCRIPTION AND IMPLICATIONS?

The label here specifies what a serving is (2/3 cup) and how many grams are contained in each serving (55 grams). Since this is a cereal, it shows how many calories you get with each serving when skim milk is added. The breakdown of the nutrients and minerals is listed and shows the amount of each in milligrams and grams and the percent of the recommended daily value is shown for the cereal with and without milk. Note that fat and carbohydrates are given as totals with the amounts of simple sugars and fiber indicated. It is important for people with diabetes to develop complete familiarity with the contents of such labels in order to monitor their overall food intake and calorie counts.

In summary, the key to a healthy lifestyle begins with good nutrition. It is important for you and your family to begin eating a low calorie, low-fat, balanced diet with an emphasis on increasing your fruits and vegetables.

Here are some helpful hints that will help you begin to eat a more healthy diet and achieve your weight loss goals:

1. **Set a reasonable weight loss goal.** Focus on dietary and exercise goals that will give you long-term, sustained weight loss.

2. **Your weight loss goal should be to reduce your body weight by 10 percent from where you started.** A weight loss goal should be about 1 to 2 pounds per week for a period of 6 months. Try to decrease your current dietary intake by 500-1000 calories per day to lose 1-2 pounds per week. In order to control your weight you should:

    a) Reduce intake of high fat foods such as fried foods, gravies, salad dressing and other fats.

    b) Control portion sizes.

3. **Eat a well-balanced diet.**

    a) Plan to eat meals 4-5 hours apart or have a snack if your meal will be delayed.

    b) Include a variety of foods according to your meal plan.

    c) Distribute foods evenly throughout the day.

4. **Eat at least five servings of fruits and vegetables a day.** Here are some suggestions to help you eat more servings of fruits and vegetables.

    a) Buy frozen, dried and fresh fruits and vegetables.

    b) Keep a fruit bowl, carrots or raisins near you at all times.

      c) Add berries or sliced fresh fruit to your breakfast cereal.

      d) Enjoy 1/2-3/4 cup of 100% fruit juice every morning.

      e) Add thinly grated carrots or zucchini to soups, sauces and casseroles for a light, sweet taste and added nutrient value.

      f) Choose fruit for dessert. Top low-fat yogurt or sherbet with berries.

5. **Eat high-fiber foods, aiming for a total fiber intake of 25-30 grams per day.**

6. **Limit fat.**

      a) Limit saturated fats such as butter, lard, whole milk, cream cheese, and fatty meats. Use skim or 1 percent milk.

      b) Control amount of fat: trim the fat from meat and remove the skin from chicken. When eating meat, poultry, or fish, limit your portion to 2 or 3 ounces (the size of the palm of your hand).

      c) Replace saturated fats with vegetable oil.

7. **If you have high blood pressure you need to decrease your salt intake to 2400 mg of sodium per day.**

8. **Use low-fat cooking techniques like grilling, broiling, baking and steaming. Avoid fried foods.**

Table 9. Exchange list. (Each item listed is one serving)

STARCH/BREADS

Starch -1 serving – 80 calories
Cereal / Beans / Grains / Pasta
Cereal (cooked) ½ cup
Beans (cooked or canned) 1/3 cup
Rice (cooked) 1/3 cup
Pasta (cooked) ½ cup

Breads – 1 serving – 80 calories
Bagel or English Muffin ½ or 1 oz.
Bread (slice or roll) 1 oz.
Crackers, snack 4-5
Graham crackers 3 squares
Hamburger or hot dog bun ½ or 1 oz.
Popcorn (plain, unbuttered) 3 cups

FRUIT

Fruit – 1 serving 60 calories	Banana (medium) ½
Cherries 12	Canned fruit in juice or water ½ cup
Apple (raw – 2" across)	Cranberry, grape or prune juice 1/3 cup
Grapes 12-15	Apple, orange or grapefruit juice ½ cup
Dried Fruit ¼ cup	

FREE FOODS HAVE LESS THAN 20 CALORIES AND HAVE VERY LITTLE AFFECT ON YOUR BLOOD SUGAR

Drink Mixes	Tea
Mineral water	Herbs
Gelatin desserts	Mustard
Sugar substitutes	Vinegar
Garlic or garlic powder	Salsa

Club soda – (Note: avoid if you have high blood pressure)

Table 10. Exchange list. (Each item listed is one serving)

MILK/DAIRY PRODUCTS

Milk – 1 serving = 90-100 calories
Low-fat or non-fat milk 8 oz.
Low-fat or non-fat buttermilk 8 oz.
Yogurt (non-fat plain or artificially sweetened) 8 oz.
Hot cocoa mix (artificially sweetened) 1 envelope

MEATS/MEAT SUBSTITUTES

Lean Meats/Meat Substitutes – 1 serving – 35-55 calories
Cheese (1-3 grams of fat) 1 oz.
Chicken (white, no skin) 1 oz.
Cottage Cheese ¼ cup
Fish (tuna, cod, flounder) 1 oz.
Lean beef (flank, round, sirloin) 1 oz.
Turkey (white, no skin) 1 oz.
Medium/High-fat Meats – 1 serving 75-100 calories
Beef 1 oz.
Chitterlings 1 oz.
Chicken (dark meat, no skin) 1 oz.
Eggs 1
Pork (spareribs, barbecue, chops, cutlets) 1 oz.
Sausage 1 oz.
Weiners 1 oz.

FATS – 1 SERVING – 5 GRAMS FAT, 45 CALORIES

Avocado (4" across) 1/8
Bacon 1 slice
Oil 1 tsp
Butter 1 tsp
Pesto Sauce 2 tsp
Salad Dressing (reduced calorie) 2 Tbsp
Cream (light, table coffee, sour) 2 Tbsp

Non-diary creamer (dry) 4 tsp
Non-dairy creamer (liquid) 2 Tbsp
Nuts or seeds 1 Tbsp
Cream Cheese 1 Tbsp
Margarine 1 tsp
Mayonnaise 1 tsp

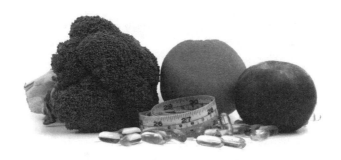

Table 11. Calories in Daily Meal Plans/ Exchanges for each Group

CALORIE MEAL PLANS (DAILY)	1,200	1,500	1,800	2,000
Starch	5	7	8	9
Fruit	3	3	4	4
Milk	2	2	3	3
Vegetables	2	2	3	4
Meats/Meat Substitutes	4	4	6	6
Fat	3	4	4	5

Table 12. Sample Menus for Each Calorie Level

1,200 CALORIES	1,200 SAMPLE MENU	1,500 CALORIES	1,800 CALORIES	2,000 CALORIES
Breakfast 1 Starch 1 Fruit 1 Milk	English muffin ½ Banana (medium) ½ Hot Cocoa Mix (artificially sweetened) 1 envelope	Add 1 starch	Add 1 Starch	Add 1 Starch 1 Fat
Lunch 1 Starch 2 Meat 1 Vegetable 1 Fruit 1 Fat	1 wheat roll 1 oz. Chicken 1 oz. Cheese 1 oz. Beans Apple (raw – 2" across) Salad dressing (reduced calorie) 2 Tbsp	1 Starch	1 Starch 1 Meat 1 Milk	1 Starch 1 Milk 1 Fat 1 Vegetable
Afternoon Snack Nothing			1 Starch	1 Starch
Dinner 2 Starch 2 Meat 1 Vegetable 1 Fruit 2 Fat	Rice 1/3 cup Peas (cooked) ½ cup Turkey 2 oz. Onions Butter 1 tsp Oil 1 tsp Canned fruit in juice ½ cup			1 Starch
Evening Snack 1 Starch 1 Milk	Low-fat or nonfat milk 8 oz. Popcorn 3 cups			

Table 13. Glycemic Index

Cake	90	Waffles	109
Doughnut	108	All Bran Cereal	60
Oat Bran	50	Special K Cereal	77
Cocoa Puffs	110	Brown Rice	79
Oatmeal Cookies	79	White Rice	126
Apple	52	Banana	78
Orange Juice	74	Macaroni & Cheese	92
Orange	62	Carrots	101
French Fries	107	Sweet Potato	77

Note: The higher the number, the faster the blood sugar rises after eating this item.

Test Your Knowledge

Diabetes and Nutrition

1. Obesity is a problem in the United States. Over 60% of Americans are considered overweight.

> TRUE FALSE

2. The two most popular food management programs for people with diabetes are carbohydrate counting and the exchange system. With the exchange system, every food on the list has about the same amount of carbohydrates, protein, fat and calories .

> TRUE FALSE

3. Food items that are high in carbohydrate content include:

   a) Desserts
   b) Jams and jellies
   c) Pasta, potatoes and rice
   d) Starchy vegetables

   1) a,b,c
   2) a,c
   3) b,d
   4) all of the above
   5) none of the above

4. Proteins and carbohydrates both provide 4 calories of energy per gram.

> TRUE FALSE

Test Your Knowledge

Diabetes and Nutrition

5. Fats are a concentrated energy source. Fat provides more than 2 times the calories you get from carbohydrates.

        TRUE   FALSE

6. If your physician agrees, alcohol can be included in a diabetes meal plan. Alcohol

    a) Provides calories but has no nutritional value
    b) Should be mixed with diabetes medications
    c) Can dramatically lower blood sugar when a person is on insulin
    d) Can be used with metformin

    1) a,b,c
    2) a,c
    3) b,d
    4) all of the above

7. Reading nutrition labels is very important since it provides information on ingredients, serving size, calories per serving and nutrient information. If you are having wide swings in your blood consider:

    a) Increasing your carbohydrate and adding fiber
    b) Decreasing your carbohydrate and adding fat
    c) Decreasing your carbohydrate and adding protein
    d) Decreasing your carbohydrate and adding fiber

    1) a,b,c
    2) a,c
    3) b,d
    4) d only

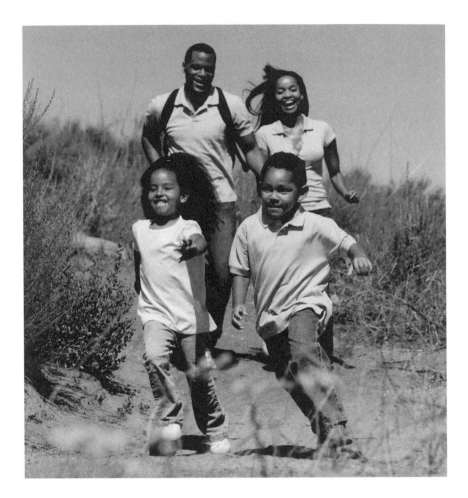

Obesity and Exercise

Many of you are thinking about starting an exercise program. The commitment to exercise will require both time and effort. You must have patience and not expect instant results. If you try to do too much too soon your chances of failure are increased. In this section, we will try to give you some basic information regarding exercise and physical fitness. The main reason that you need to incorporate exercise into your daily routine is to decrease your chances of becoming overweight or obese.

Obesity is a life-threatening disease affecting 34% of adults

Section 2 - Diabetes Management

in the U.S. Nearly 67% of adults in the U.S. are either overweight or obese. Between 2000 and 2005, obesity (BMI ≥30) increased by 24%, morbid obesity (BMI ≥ 40) increased by 50% and super obesity (BMI ≥ 50) increased by 75%. As of 2006, 11% of preschoolers ages 2 to 5, 15% of children ages 6 to 11 and 18% of adolescents ages 12 to 19 are over-weight. Overweight adolescents have a 70% chance of becoming over-weight or obese adults. This increases to 80% if one or more parent is overweight or obese. The increases in obesity were evident regardless of sex, age, race, and educational status.

The obesity epidemic is due to less physical activity and more calories being consumed than used. We are eating more pre-packaged foods and more "fast foods," and drinking more high calorie drinks. Our portion size has also increased, therefore we consume more calories during our meals and snacks. The increase in calories means increased energy intake causing weight gain.

According to the report from the Office of Minority Health, African American women have the highest rates of being overweight or obese compared to other groups in the U.S. About four out of five African American women are overweight or obese. In 2009, African Americans were 1.5 times as likely to be obese as Non- Hispanic Whites. In 2009, African American women were 60% more likely to be obese than Non-Hispanic White women. In 2007-2008, African American children were 30% as likely to be overweight than Non-Hispanic Whites. Reasons for the increase in obesity in African Americans can be attributed to increased fat consumption and less physical activity.

How is obesity measured?

Obesity is measured using the BMI (Body Mass Index) or waist circumference. BMI is a number that shows body weight adjusted for height. BMI can be calculated with simple math using inches and pounds, or meters and kilograms. For adults aged 20 years or older, BMI falls into one of these categories: underweight, normal, overweight, or obese.

Table 14. Categories of Body Mass Index

BMI (kg/m²)	Weight Status
Below 18.5	Underweight
18.5 – 24.9	Normal
25.0 – 29.9	Overweight
30.0 and Above	Obese

BMI correlates with the amount of body fat. The relation between the percent body fat and BMI differs with age and gender. For example, women are more likely to have a higher percent of body fat than men for the same BMI. The goal is to keep your BMI less than 25 kg/m². Table 14 provides you with your BMI based on your height and weight in pounds.

Whatever your BMI, talk to your health care provider to see if you are at an increased risk for disease and if you should lose weight. Even a small weight loss (just 7-10% of your current weight) may help to lower the risk of disease.

Waist circumference is a common measure used to assess abdominal fat content. There is evidence that excess body fat in the abdomen, is an independent predictor of risk factors for many chronic diseases including diabetes and heart disease.

Undesirable waist circumferences differ for men and women

- Men are at risk if they have a waist measurement greater than 40 inches (102 cm)
- Women are at risk if they have a waist measurement greater than 35 inches (88 cm)

It is important that you work to achieve your goal for BMI and/or waist circumference in order to reduce your risk for chronic diseases and complications later in life.

Being Overweight or Obesity can Cause Problems

Overweight and obese individuals (BMI of 25 and above) are at increased risk for many chronic diseases and conditions.

Examples include:

- High blood cholesterol
- High blood pressure, hypertension – 50 million people
- Diabetes – (18 million people with diabetes (Type 1 and Type 2)
- Coronary heart disease – 13.5 million people
- Angina pectoris (Chest pain due to lack of oxygen to the heart)
- Congestive heart failure (Heart cannot pump out blood, as a result blood backs up in the heart).
- Stroke (Brain attack due to lack of oxygen to the brain)
- Problems with the Gall Bladder and Gallstones
- Gout
- Osteoarthritis
- Obstructive sleep apnea and respiratory problems
- Some types of cancer (such as endometrial, breast, prostate, and colon)
- Complications of pregnancy
- Poor female reproductive health (such as menstrual irregularities, infertility, irregular ovulation)

- Bladder control problems (such as stress incontinence)
- Psychological disorders (such as depression, eating disorders, distorted body image, and low self esteem).

Numerous studies have shown that weight loss can decrease the risk of developing the diseases/conditions mentioned above. The best way to lose weight or not to gain weight is proper nutrition and exercise.

Physical Activity / Exercise

More than 60 percent of U.S. adults do not engage in the recommended amount of activity. Approximately 25 percent of U.S. adults are not active at all. Physical inactivity is more common among:

- **Women than men.**
- **African American and Hispanic** adults than whites.
- **Older than younger adults.**
- **Less affluent** than more affluent people.

Based upon years of research we now know that increasing our physical activity level generally promotes good health and fewer disabilities later in life. Learning to incorporate exercise into your daily routine at home and at work will help you to live a longer and healthier life. The more exercise you get the better you will feel. The most important aspect to a successful exercise routine is that you must do it regularly (rain or shine). We tend to make excuses why we cannot find the time to exercise.

Some of the common excuses include:

"I don't have the time"

"I am too old to exercise"

"I need special clothing to exercise"

"I have joint pain due to arthritis"

"People at the gym will think I am fat"

"I cannot afford a gym membership"

"I don't know how to exercise"

"I don't want to take time away from my family"

"I don't like to sweat"

"It will mess up my hair"

The reality is that you are never too old to exercise. It is not necessary for you to purchase an expensive gym membership or buy special clothes. Simply walking and incorporating more activity into your daily life can improve your fitness level.

There are many benefits to exercise. They include:

- Aerobic exercise burns fat and calories
- Anaerobic Exercise -Weight training increases muscle tissue which raises metabolic rate
- Reduces blood pressure
- Reduces LDL-C (Bad Cholesterol) and raises HDL-C (Good) Cholesterol
- Decreases blood sugar levels
- Improves insulin sensitivity
- Relieves some types of stress and depression
- Reduces the intensity of menopause and premenstrual symptoms
- Improves body composition
- Reduces the craving for tobacco
- Improves exercise capacity and stamina
- Increases blood fibrinolytic capacity (prevents blood clots, which can cause a heart attack or stroke)
- Slows the process of aging

Components of an exercise prescription

Before you start exercising it is important to check with your health care provider. If you have certain medical conditions (diabetes and the presence of diabetic complications, heart failure, high blood pressure, coronary heart disease, etc.) exercise can increase your risk of serious injury. Your health care provider may give you a special test to make sure that you can tolerate a basic exercise program. In general, exercise improves most chronic conditions. When choosing your exercise regimen pick something that you like to do that does not cause any discomfort. A mixture of weight bearing (walking, jogging) and non-weight bearing (swimming) will reduce your risk of joint injury. When deciding on your exercise routine you must select the type, duration, frequency and intensity of your exercise program.

Type or Mode of Exercise

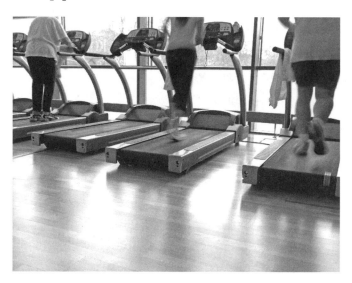

Aerobic

The American College of Sports Medicine (ACSM) defines aerobic exercise as "any activity that uses large muscle groups, can be maintained continuously, and is rhythmic in nature." It is a type of exercise that targets the heart and lungs and causes them to work harder than at rest. Some examples of aerobic exercise include:

- Walking
- Swimming
- Volleyball
- Tennis
- Bicycling
- Jumping rope
- Jogging
- Stair walking
- Ice or roller-skating
- Downhill or Cross-County skiing
- Aerobic equipment (i.e. Treadmill)
- Dancing

What is Resistance / Strength training?

Resistance or weight training involves using different muscle groups to lift weights. This type of exercise works against the forces of gravity. These exercises are not limited to lifting huge barbells, but also include, raising the legs with ankle weights attached.

What are the Benefits of Strength Training through Resistance Exercises?

There are numerous benefits to strength training regularly, particularly as you grow older. Strength training can help you to control your weight since individuals who have more muscle mass have a higher metabolic rate. Muscle is an active tissue that consumes calories while stored fat uses very little energy. Strength training can provide up to a 15% increase in metabolic rate, which is enormously helpful for weight loss and long-term weight control. Studies have shown that lifting weights two or three times a week increases strength by building muscle mass and bone density. It can be very powerful in reducing the signs and symptoms of numerous diseases and chronic conditions, among them:

Arthritis – One study found strength training decreased pain by 43%, increased muscle strength and general physical performance, improved the clinical signs and symptoms of the disease, and decreased disability.

Diabetes – Clinical studies have shown that adding resistance training to an established exercise routine can produce dramatic improvements in glucose control that are comparable to taking diabetes medication. People with diabetes that participate in resistance training are stronger, gained muscle, lose body fat, and have less depression.

Osteoporosis - Post-menopausal women can lose 1-2% of their bone mass annually. Resistance training can increase bone density and reduces the risk for fractures among women aged 50-70.

Depression - Strength training provides similar improvements in depression as anti-depressant medications. Currently, it is not known if this is because people feel better when they are stronger or if strength training produces a helpful biochemical change in the brain. It is most likely a combination of the two.

Insomnia - People who exercise regularly enjoy improved sleep quality. They fall asleep more quickly, sleep more deeply, awaken less often, and sleep longer.

Heart Disease – The risk of heart disease is lower when the body is leaner. One study found that cardiac patients gained not only strength and flexibility but also aerobic capacity when strength training was done three times a week as part of their rehabilitation program.

Duration and Frequency of Exercise

The new exercise guidelines recommend the following:

Two hours and 30 minutes (150 minutes) of moderate intensity aerobic activity every week. Over time we would like you to increase to 5 hours (300 minutes) per week. This 150 minute recommendation is based on the information obtained from the Diabetes Prevention Program. In that study, participants that exercised, 150 minutes per week and ate a low fat diet were able to decrease their risk of getting diabetes by 58%. Doing your exercise in short 10 minute sessions is OK. It is actually best to spread your activity out during the week.

Resistance Training – Muscle Strengthening should be done 2 or more days a week working all of the major muscle groups (legs, hips, back, abdomen, chest, shoulders and arms. Older individuals should train at least two days per week but no more than four. The average duration of the training session is 30-45 minutes.

Intensity

Exercise can be categorized as low, moderate and high intensity. Low intensity exercise is < 50% of maximum heart rate (MHR). Moderate intensity exercise is 50-70% of MHR. High intensity exercise is >90% of MHR. Measuring your heart rate (beats per minute) can tell you how hard your heart is working and is a good method for measuring the intensity of your exercise. The goal is to raise your heart rate to a certain level and keep it there for at least 20 minutes. The heart rate you maintain is called your target heart rate. You can check your heart rate by counting your pulse for 15 seconds and multiplying the beats by 4.

When you're just beginning an exercise program, shoot for the low intensity (50% MHR). As your fitness improves, you can exercise harder to get your heart rate closer to the high intensity level of 90% MHR.

Getting Started

Warm-up – Start every workout with a 5-10 minute warm-up to make your muscles and joints more flexible. Spend 5-10 minutes of with light calisthenics and stretching exercises. Use low intensity movement, like, knee lifts, walking, arm circles or trunk rotations.

Exercise Routine – include a minimum of two 30-minute sessions each week of resistance training of all the major muscle groups. Start out with one set of each exercise 8-10 repetitions. The goal would be to work your way up to 3 sets of each exercise with 10-15 repetitions. Aerobic exercise should be a minimum of three 30-minute sessions each week with a goal of 45-60 minutes every day.

Cool Down – a minimum of 5-10 minutes of slow walking, low-level exercise, combined with stretching.

In summary, increasing your daily physical activity and incorporating exercise into your daily life can improve your health and decrease your risk of chronic diseases. Remember to make exercise fun, work it into your daily calendar, exercise with a partner and most of all, don't get discouraged. It can take weeks or even months before you notice a physical difference. However, after a day or two, you will notice an improvement in mood and an increase in your level of energy.

Test Your Knowledge
Obesity and Exercise

1. The obesity epidemic in the United States is due to:

   a) More physical activity, high caloric drinks, more fast foods and larger portions
   b) Less physical activity, high caloric drinks, more fast foods and smaller portions
   c) More physical activity, low caloric drinks, more fast foods and smaller portions
   d) Less physical activity, high caloric drinks, more fast foods and larger portions

2. African Americans and Latinos have higher rates of obesity compared to other ethnic groups.

   TRUE   FALSE

3. Obesity can increase your risk for:

   a) Heart Attacks
   b) High Blood Pressure
   c) Cancer
   d) Stroke

   1) a,b,c
   2) a,c
   3) b,d
   4) all of the above
   5) none of the above

Test Your Knowledge

Obesity and Exercise

4. The benefits of exercise include:

   a) Reducing blood pressure values
   b) Decreasing stress and slowing aging
   c) Improving insulin sensitivity
   d) Raising "good" cholesterol (HDL)

   1) a,b,c
   2) a,c
   3) b,d
   4) all of the above

5. Aerobic exercise is defined as an activity that uses the larger muscle groups, is continuous and rhythmic. Examples of aerobic exercise include:

   a) Walking, swimming, dancing, weight lifting
   b) Jogging, jumping rope, stair walking, rollerskating
   c) Volleyball, tennis, bicycling, weight lifting
   d) Leg raises with weights, baseball, walking, and basketball

6. Increasing daily activity can improve your overall health. Your exercise goals should be two 30-minute sessions of resistance training exercises each week and 45-60 minutes of aerobic exercise each day.

   TRUE   FALSE

Management of Diabetes with Medication

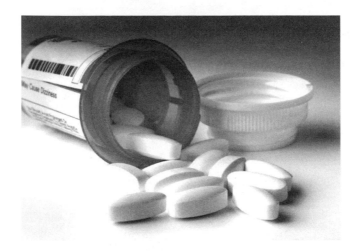

What kind of medications can my health care provider give me for my diabetes?

People with Type 2 diabetes may have to take medications prescribed by their health care provider when both meal planning and exercise do not control their diabetes.

In people with Type 2, either the pancreas is not producing enough insulin or the body is not responding to the insulin produced. The latter is a condition called insulin resistance. In order for oral antidiabetic pills to work, patients must have insulin present in their body. Remember, in Type 1 patients there is an absolute lack of insulin, therefore oral antidiabetic pills will not work. Insulin is the drug of choice for Type 1 patients with diabetes.

Currently, there are a total of nine classes of antidiabetic medications. And others are under development at the time of this writing. Each class distinguishes itself from the other by the way in which they lower blood glucose. Of these antidiabetic medications, six are for oral use (pill form, to be taken by mouth) and three are injectables. Insulin is one type of the injectables.

Oral Antidiabetic Medications (Pills)

Insulin Secreting Agents (Oral Hypoglycemics)

Sulfonylurea Class - There are several agents in this class, which include, glyburide (Micronase®), glipizide (Glucotrol®), glimepiride (Amaryl®). These help the pancreas to secrete insulin.

Meglitinide Class - Repaglinide (Prandin®) and nateglinide (Starlix®) also help the pancreas to secrete more insulin, these agents are especially effective for lowering blood glucose levels after a meal.

Insulin Sensitizers

Thiazolidinedione Class - The thiazolidinediones, (pioglitazine (Actos®) and rosiglitazone (Avandia®) decreases insulin resistance in the muscle. This way, when insulin brings the glucose to the tissue, the glucose is successfully taken up by the tissue for energy use or storage. They may also help reduce the accumulation of fat in the liver of patients with type 2 diabetes and reduce the tendency for development of atherosclerosis. Unfortunately, these agents are beginning to experince limitations on their use.

Biguanide Class - The only member of this class available in the U.S. is metformin (Glucophage®). Metformin works to increase the tissue sensitivity to insulin, thereby increasing the uptake of the glucose. It also reduces the amount of glucose made by the liver.

Alpha Glucosidase Inhibitor Class

Acarbose (Precose®), miglitol (Glyset®) are included in this class. People with diabetes have even higher than normal levels of blood sugar after eating; these are known as "spikes". The alpha glucosidase inhibitors slow the body's digestion of sugars and starches after eating a meal, and hence help prevent spikes.

Dipeptidyl Peptidase-IV (DPP-IV) Inhibitor Class

There are currently three available agents in this class, Sitagliptin (Januvia®), Saxagliptin (Onglyza®) and Linagliptin (Tradjenta®). These agents increase insulin secretion. They stop the liver from making glucose. Sitagliptin, Saxagliptin and Linagliptin halt the action of DPP-IV from destroying certain hormones (incretin hormones). The prolonged action of the incretin hormones help to release insulin from the pancreas thereby lowering glucose levels. Other agents in this class that are in use or under development include vildagliptin and alogliptin.

Injectable Antidiabetic Medications

Until recently, the only injectable medication (given by injection using a syringe) for the treatment of diabetes was insulin. In the past few years we now have two new injectable medications that are used in the treatment of diabetes.

Amylin Analog Class

Pramlintide (Symlin®). Injectable, pramlintide, is indicated for Type 1 and Type 2 diabetics who use mealtime insulin. Our bodies secrete amylin, along with insulin after a meal. However, in people with diabetes there is a shortage of amylin. Pramlintide is a man-made form of amylin, which mimics the action of amylin. Pramlintide, through a variety of mechanisms, helps to reduce the rise in glucose levels after a meal, by inhibiting glucagon. Glucagon causes the liver to make glucose by providing a feeling of fullness. Pramlintide helps to reduce food intake and promotes weight loss. Patients should be advised to reduce the pre-meal insulin dose by 50% when taking this agent. Always follow the advice of your personal health care provider pertaining to your insulin dosing.

Incretin Mimetic Class

Incretin mimetics are a new class of drugs which mimic the hormone GLP-1 (glucagon like peptide 1) and GIP (gastric inhibitory peptide). These hormones have been found to increase insulin release in response to glucose stimulation; stop the liver from making glucose, by inhibiting glucagon secretion; and slow digestion. Studies have shown that slowing the digestion can actually help in controlling diabetes by reducing the levels of post meal glucose. The effect on Glucagon is important since Glucagon causes the liver to make glucose during the night and is why many people with diabetes have high morning blood sugars. The most noteworthy fact about these agents is their ability to cause significant weight loss, as much as 30 pounds in some patients. Their weight loss effect is due to their ability to decrease hunger.

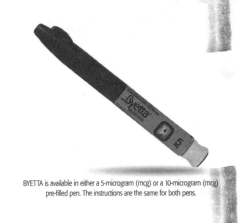

BYETTA is available in either a 5-microgram (mcg) or a 10-microgram (mcg) pre-filled pen. The instructions are the same for both pens.

Exenatide (Byetta®), an injectable agent, synthetic version of a hormone exendin-4 that was found in the saliva of the Gila monster. Gila monsters eat infrequently, and exendin-4 in the saliva helps them digest meals slowly over time.

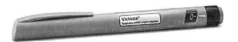

Liraglutide (Victoza®), is a synthetic injectable agent that works like the body's own human glucagon-like peptide (GLP-1). Liraglutide attaches to the GLP-1 receptors in the intestine and stays around in the body for a much longer time then own GLP-1 hormone. Liraglutide is used as an add on therapy to diet and exercise from the treatment of type 2 diabetes. It works by increasing insulin release from the pancreas when the blood sugar levels are elevated. Liraglutide also decreases glucagon secretion from the pancreas and slows down the emptying of the stomach. This drug is usually prescribed after you have been on metformin and another oral agent with no success. Liraglutide is not a substitute for insulin therapy. Liraglutide is similar to Exenatide, which was the first GLP-1 agonist in its class to be indicated for the treatment of adult patients with type 2 diabetes mellitus. Both drugs should not be used for the treatment of diabetic ketoacidosis..

Both Exenatide and Liraglutide are recommended for use only in patients with Type 2 diabetes who are already receiving Metformin, a Sulfonylurea, or both and are not at their blood glucose goal. When these agents are added to Metformin therapy, the current dose of Metformin can be continued without adjustment. However, when Incretin Mimetics are added to Sulfonylurea therapy, a reduction in the dose of Sulfonylurea should be considered to prevent hypoglycemia.

Can I control my diabetes with drug?

It is important to understand that most patients with diabetes will require at least two to three medications to control their blood sugar and get to goal. You will need to take a combination of medications that work by different mechanisms of action. In most cases, Metformin is the drug of choice for patients that have type 2 diabetes. Most of the current diabetes guidelines recommend starting with Metforim. Sulfonlyureas like Glimepiride or Glipizide are still used as first line therapy especially in those patients that have high blood sugars (above 250mg/dL). The increased rate of low blood sugar reactions and weight gain limit the use of the Sulfonylureas. If you blood sugar is not controlled on one drug (blood sugar goal is 90-130mg/dL) then your doctor will need to add a second oral medication or an injectable drug like Byetta® or Victoza®. If you are not able to get your A1C to 7% or less on these agents your doctor may need to start insulin therapy.

Insulin Injections

Why does my health care provider tell me I need insulin?

As the "housekeeper" of the nutrients you eat, insulin is necessary for your body to work properly. It helps the body to lower the amount of glucose in the blood, allows the body to use blood glucose for energy, and helps store the glucose for future use.

You may need daily insulin shots to control your blood glucose. If you have Type 1 diabetes, you will need to use insulin for the rest of your life. In patients with Type 2 diabetes, insulin can be added to most oral medications. Recent medical advances make giving insulin very easy.

What are the different types of insulin?

There are 3 important things to know about your insulin:

- Class of insulin (both source and type).
- How much to use.
- When to administer.

When you buy your insulin, you should make sure that you always receive the same kind and brand of insulin as prescribed by your health care provider. It's a good idea to check the expiration date as well.

In the past, pigs and cows were the only available sources of insulin. Now drug companies can use other methods to manufacture insulin that is almost identical to the insulin made by the human body. This is called human insulin.

There are now "new" synthetic insulins that are either ultra-fast acting or ultra-slow acting. These new insulins are called "insulin analogs" and are designed to better mimic your body's own insulin. The rapid acting insulin analogs; lispro (Humalog®), aspart (Novolog®), glulisine (Apidra®) can be injected as late as 5 minutes prior to a meal. The long-acting analogs; glargine (Lantus®), detemir (Levemir®) can be injected once daily during mornings, bedtime or at some other time along with your oral medications to provide smoother and tighter control of your blood sugar.

The insulin analogs tend to cause fewer low-blood sugar reactions due to the way they work in the body. Insulin also differs in the time that it takes to work. Regardless of the source, there are five available types of insulin: lispro and aspart (rapid-acting), human regular (short acting); NPH, lente (intermediate-acting); ultralente (long-acting), and glargine/detemir (ultra-long-acting). Your health care provider may have you use two types of insulin in a single shot. If so, ask your health care provider, pharmacist, or nurse how to mix the two types together. Insulin glargine has to be given as a separate shot and not mixed with other insulin due to the difference in pH.

In order to achieve "good" blood sugar control most people with Type 1 diabetes will rarely require less than two injections a day. People with Type 2 diabetes either are receiving one shot a day of insulin along with their oral medicines or multiple shots a day. It is important that you do not avoid taking insulin if your health care provider feels you need it, especially if you are not at your goal fasting blood sugar (goal = 90-130 mg/dL). Delaying the use of insulin may increase your chance of having the long-term complications of diabetes. Your physician should instruct you on how much insulin to use and when to use it.

Can you purchase regular and intermediate acting insulin in the same bottle?

Most patients on insulin need a combination of both regular/rapid-acting an intermediate or long-acting insulin to adequately control their blood sugar. There are mixtures of NPH (intermediate insulin) and regular insulin (short-acting)/rapid acting that are available from the manufacturer. See Table 16. These mixtures remain stable for one month at room temperature or for three months refrigerated. Pre-mixed insulin is also available in pre-filled syringes (insulin pens). Patients that have vision problems, hand tremors, arthritis or have difficulty drawing up insulin into the syringe, may find that pre-mixed insulin is easier to use. Ask your health care provider if you are a potential candidate for pre-mixed insulin.

What does a bottle of insulin look like?

Insulin comes in two strengths (100 or 500 units per milliliter). You should look at the insulin bottle before each use. Examine the insulin for any changes. If the insulin looks lumpy, frosted, flaky, or if there are any changes in color, do not use it without your health care provider's permission. Be aware that some types of insulin are normally cloudy. Usually intermediate and long acting insulins are cloudy. An exception is with insulin glargine, an ultra long-acting insulin that is clear in color and not cloudy due to the different pH of the product. Store unopened insulin bottles in the refrigerator. You may keep opened insulin bottles out of the refrigerator at room temperature. However, you should throw away any insulin bottle that has been out of the refrigerator for more than thirty (30) days.

What does an insulin syringe look like?

Insulin syringes are smaller than the kind the health care provider or nurse uses for antibiotic or flu shots. Although insulin syringes can hold up to 1 milliliter of insulin, your health care provider will instruct you to draw up only a small amount for use. The insulin syringes come in different sizes based on the amount of insulin you use per shot. The 1 milliliter (also known as cc) syringe are for those people who need up to 100 units of insulin. If you are using less insulin per shot you may want to consider using the ¼ cc, 3/10 cc or ½ cc syringe. It is important that you match your insulin dosage to your syringe. For example if you are taking 30 units or less of insulin, you would use the 3/10 cc syringe. The ½ cc syringe should be used if you are taking 50 units or less of insulin per shot. Most insulin syringe manufacturers do not recommend that you re-use the syringes. Re-use of insulin syringes may lead to discomfort due to needle dullness, possible infection or tissue damage. There are many people with diabetes that re-use their syringes without any problems. If you want to re-use your syringes you should discuss this practice with your health care provider, diabetes educator or pharmacist. If you re-use the syringe make sure you recap the needle and wipe the needle off with alcohol prior to injecting the needle into your skin.

How do I prepare my insulin shot?

It is very important for you to carefully prepare your insulin shot. You may want to follow these steps when getting your insulin shot ready:

Step 1 — Before each insulin shot, wash your hands with soap and water.

Step 2 — Wipe the top of the insulin bottle with an unused alcohol pad.

Step 3 — Gently roll the bottle between the palms of your hands to mix the insulin.

Step 4 — Draw an amount of air equal to your insulin dose into the syringe, stick the needle into the insulin bottle and inject the air into the insulin bottle. (For example, if your insulin dose is 25 units, that equals 0.25 ml - draw 0.25 ml of air into the syringe and inject it into the bottle.)

Step 5 — With the syringe still in the insulin bottle, invert the bottle of insulin and withdraw the correct amount of insulin into the syringe.

Step 6 — If you are mixing two kinds of insulin, draw the short-acting insulin first and the long or intermediate-acting insulin second. In order to do this, one must draw the total amount of units needed of air (short acting + long acting) into the syringe. Inject the amount of air equivalent to the dose of the long acting FIRST in the long vacting insulin bottle. DO NOT TAKE ANY OF THE LONG ACTING INSULIN OUT OF THE BOTTLE. After putting air in the long acting bottle take the syringe out of the bottle. THEN inject air equal to the dose of the short acting insulin into the short acting insulin bottle. While needle is still in the bottle, turn the bottle upside down and withdraw the dose required of the short acting insulin. Then stick the needle in the long acting bottle of insulin, turn bottle upside down and withdraw the dose needed of the long acting insulin.

Step 7 — Before injecting, look at the syringe and remove any bubbles by tapping or flicking your finger against the side of the syringe.

Figure 2

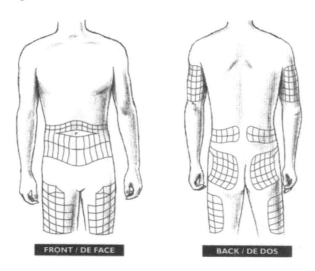

FRONT / DE FACE   BACK / DE DOS

Where do I inject my insulin?

Inject insulin shots underneath the skin, but not into a muscle or blood vessel. If you inject cloudy insulin into a muscle it may cause damage and inflammation (swelling). If you inject clear insulin into a blood vessel, the uptake may be too rapid and may cause hypoglycemia. For small children, it may be necessary to inject the insulin at an angle to avoid shooting the insulin into a muscle. For adults with diabetes, pinch a fold of skin and inject the insulin straight into the fold.

Give insulin shots either in the upper arm, the front/side of the thigh, the buttocks, or the stomach area (except the 2-inch area around the belly button - Figure 2). You should not use the same area of skin for each shot, but use the same part of the body every time you inject insulin. For example, if you inject insulin into your stomach, move to a different area of the stomach and do not change to the thigh or arm the next time for your insulin shot.

What do I do if the insulin shot hurts too much?

If you feel pain or if blood appears where you injected the insulin, you should press down on the affected area for 5 to 8 seconds without rubbing the skin. Talk to your health care provider or nurse if your skin bleeds, bruises, or gets sore or red in the place where you gave your insulin shot. Some of the newer insulin analogs (glargine) can cause pain at the site of injection even with a properly administered injection. The pain on injection from glargine usually improves with time. If you are experiencing a lot of pain when you inject, let your health care provider know.

How do I know how much insulin to give to myself?

The amount of insulin that you need depends on how high or low your blood glucose is throughout the day. There are many things that can change how well your body uses insulin. Exercise, stress, food and illness all may have an effect on the amount of insulin that you need. Therefore, you may need to check your blood glucose several times throughout the day to determine the correct amount of insulin needed.

If your blood glucose is too high after measuring, you will need to give yourself extra insulin according to your health care provider's directions. If your blood glucose is too low, you need to eat or drink something that contains glucose unless you feel like falling asleep. In that case, someone who knows that you have diabetes needs to contact a health care provider for help as soon as possible. If you fall asleep, this person should not give you any food or drink by mouth or you may choke.

It is very important for you to follow your health care provider's instructions on when and how to properly use insulin shots. The time course of action of any insulin may vary in different individuals, or at different times in the same individual. Because of this variation, the time period indicated here should be considered general guidelines only.

Table 15. Comparison of Human Insulin and Analogues

Insulin Preparations	Onset of Action	Peak Time	Duration of Action
Lispro/Aspart/ Glulisine	5 - 15 minutes	1 - 2 hours	3 - 4 hours
Human Regular	30 - 60 minutes	2 - 3 hours	3 - 6 hours
Human NPH	2 - 4 hours	4 - 10 hours	
Detemir	40 minutes- 2 hrs	Unpredictable	10 - 16 hrs
Glargine	2 - 4 hours	Flat (no peak)	20 - 24 hrs

What are insulin mixtures (Premixed insulin)?

Since most people use both rapid or short acting insulin and an intermediate acting insulin, several of the insulin manufacturers have combined NPH and regular (or rapid acting insulin) into the same syringe. Most premixed insulins are available in prefilled insulin pens, which are portable. The insulin pens also are very accurate since you can dial in the number of units required for each injection instead of having to draw up the insulin into a syringe from a bottle. Table 15 provides a listing of the various insulin mixtures available on the market.

Table 16. Comparison of Premixed Insulins

Premixed Insulin Preparations	Brand Name	Form	Cloudy or Clear
50% lispro protamine, 50% insulin lispro	Humalog Mix 50/50	Analog	Cloudy
70% NPH / 30% regular	Humulin 70/30	Human	Cloudy
70% NPH/30% regular	Novolin 70/30	Human	Cloudy
75% lispro protamine/NPL 25% lispro	Humalog Mix 75/25	Analog	Cloudy
70% aspart protamine / 30% aspart	NovoLog Mix 70/30	Analog	Cloudy

What are insulin injection devices?

Insulin injection devices, also known as "insulin pens," are mechanical instruments that are used to give insulin injections. The pens have cartridges filled with insulin. The insulin cartridges available on the market contain regular insulin, intermediate-acting insulin, or a fixed combination of both regular and intermediate.

The benefits of the insulin pens are:

- **Accurate dosing** – no measuring or drawing up the insulin. Simply dial in the number of insulin units required.
- **Convenience** – insulin and syringes combined in a "pocket-size" pen.
- **Painless injection** – needles are microfine (short and thin), causing essentially no pain upon injection.
- There are also devices available that provide high-speed injection of insulin through the skin with no needles required. These insulin injectors sometimes cause bruising at the site of injection. Check with your pharmacist or diabetes educator regarding the types of injection devices available and to make sure that you are obtaining "good" blood glucose control using these devices.

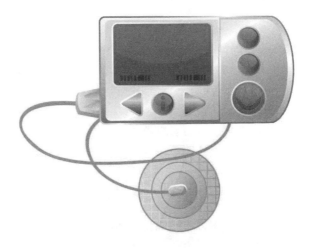

Insulin Pump Therapy

What is an insulin pump?

An insulin pump is a small, battery powered device that delivers insulin. It is about the size of a cell phone or pager. An insulin pump is another way you can get the insulin your body needs to help you take care of your diabetes.

How does an insulin pump deliver insulin?

An insulin pump uses fast-acting insulin and delivers this insulin in the following two ways:

- **Basal** – This is the insulin that your body needs continuously, throughout the day and night, to keep your glucose levels stable between meals and during sleep. The basal insulin is programmed to work automatically. Basal insulin can be delivered in different amounts for different times of the day, and can be adjusted for changes in activity. You would work with your health care provider to program the correct basal amounts.

- **Bolus** – This is the extra insulin your body needs to cover sugar and starch intake and to lower high glucose levels. Bolus insulin is not delivered automatically. Every time you need bolus insulin, you press buttons on the pump to deliver your dose. You would work with your health care provider to learn how to calculate your bolus doses.

How does an insulin pump get insulin into the body?

The pump is NOT surgically placed. An infusion set is inserted under the skin. The infusion set is attached to the pump, and the pump is worn on the outside of the body. You are taught how to insert an infusion set, and you change the infusion set every 2 – 3 days. The typical steps you would follow to fill your pump with insulin and connect yourself to the pump are listed below.

Step 1 — You fill a special cartridge with fast-acting insulin and place this cartridge into the insulin pump.

Step 2 — Next, you connect the cartridge of insulin to a piece of tubing, and this piece of tubing is connected to the infusion set.

Step 3 — You insert the infusion set into the fatty tissue just under your skin. The infusion set is inserted with a needle, similar to an insulin injection. Once the infusion set is inserted, the needle is removed and a tiny, flexible piece of tubing, called a cannula, is left under your skin.

Insulin is then "pumped" (pushed) from the cartridge, through the tubing, and then through the cannula into the fatty tissue under your skin.

Currently, there is one pump available that does not require tubing for insulin delivery. The name of this pump is Omnipod and you can find more information about this device by visiting the website www.myomnipod.com.

What are the possible benefits of using an insulin pump?

- You may improve your glucose control and reduce your risk of low glucose levels because the pump delivers insulin very precisely.
- You may experience more flexibility in your lifestyle because the pump allows you to adjust your insulin doses for changes in your sleep, meal or physical activity schedules.
- You may find an increase in convenience and privacy because the pump allows you to deliver your insulin doses by pressing buttons on the pump, instead of injecting yourself with insulin several times a day.
- You would take fewer injections because the pump infusion set is inserted once every 2 – 3 days, whereas injections of insulin are given several times a day.

Currently, most people who use insulin pumps have type 1 diabetes, but insulin pumps have also been shown to be safe and effective for people with type 2 diabetes. Insulin pumps can offer the same benefits described above to those who have type 2 diabetes.

What are some possible challenges with using an insulin pump?

- There is a risk of diabetic ketoacidosis (DKA) if the flow of insulin from the insulin pump is stopped. DKA is a serious condition that can happen when there is not enough insulin in the body.
- There is a risk of skin or infusion site problems. These problems can result from an allergic reaction to the adhesive tape, leaving the infusion set in place longer than 2 – 3 days or constantly using the same location to insert the infusion set.
- Some people find that learning how to use a new device can be overwhelming. However, you would receive training and support to help you with the transition from injections to

insulin pump therapy.

- Some people may feel bothered by being constantly attached to a medical device.
- Some people may find that out-of-pocket costs for an insulin pump can make it hard to afford this type of therapy, especially if they do not have any form of medical insurance.

What are realistic expectations with using an insulin pump?

- **An insulin pump does not check your blood glucose levels. You are still required to check your blood glucose at least four times a day.**
- An insulin pump does not automatically adjust your insulin based on your glucose levels. You need to tell the pump if you need more or less insulin based on your blood glucose readings.
- An insulin pump is not a cure for diabetes and it does not prevent high and low glucose levels by itself, but it can help to reduce the number and severity of high and low glucose readings.
- It is still very important to eat healthy foods in reasonable amounts when you use an insulin pump. An insulin pump is not a reason to eat or drink whatever you want simply because it is easy to press a few buttons on the pump to give yourself the extra insulin you need for your carbohydrates. Before starting on an insulin pump, you would learn how to count carbohydrates and how to dose your insulin to match the amount of carbohydrates (sugar and starches) that you eat.

How can I learn more about insulin pump therapy?

The companies that make insulin pumps have online resources for you to learn more about insulin pump therapy. The company names and websites are listed below:

Animas Corporation	www.animas.com
Insulet Corporation	www.myomnipod.com
Medtronic Minimed, Inc.	www.minimed.com
Roche	www.accu-chekinsulinpumps.com

A prescription is required for an insulin pump. You should talk to your health care provider if you have other questions. If your health care provider does not prescribe insulin pumps and is not able to answer your questions, consider asking your health care provider for a referral to a diabetes specialist.

Antidiabetic Medication Charts

Action: Helps the pancreas to secrete insulin

ORAL ANTIDIABETIC DRUG CLASS – SULFONYLUREAS (INSULIN SECRETING AGENTS)	Daily Dosing**		How To Take It	TAKE NOTE	TAKE ACTION
	Initial	Maximum			
First Generation				Expect to see lowering of blood glucose levels after the first dose	Due to possible hypoglycemia, and to make sure the medication is working, check your blood sugars twice daily minimal
Chlorpropamide* (Diabinase®)	100-250 mg once daily	750 mg once daily	With AM / First Meal	Hypoglycemia- can occur in all patients, mainly in patients:	Wear sunscreen and sunglasses while on these medications
Tolazamide* (Tolamide®, Tolinase®)	100-250 mg once daily	1000 (500 mg twice daily)	With AM / First Meal	-who are elderly(> 65 years of age) or have problems with their kidneys -who have implemented an exercise program and/ or reduced portion/caloric diet	Tell your provider: - if you are having more than 3 hypoglycemic reactions [< 70mg/dl per week (increase heart rate, sweating, hunger, lightheadness) your dose may have to be adjusted
Tolbutamide* (Orinase®)	1000-2000 mg once daily	3000 (1500 mg twice daily)	With Meals		
Second Generation				Can cause sensitivity to the sun	
Glyburide* (Micronase®, Diabeta®, Glynase®)	2.5-5 mg once daily	20 mg (10 mg twice daily)	With Meals		
Micronized Glyburide* (Glynase PresTab®)	1.5–3 mg once daily	12 mg (6 mg twice daily)	With Meals	Other side effects: Weight gain, constipation, rash	- if you experience rash, fever, sore throat or unusual bruising
Glipizide* (Glucotrol®)	5 mg once daily	40 mg (20 mg twice daily)	30 minutes before or with meals	The First Generation Agents are not used as commonly anymore	
Glipizide Extended Release* (Glucotrol XL®)	5 mg once daily	20 mg (10 mg twice daily)	30 minutes before or with meals	None of these agents are recommended in pregnancy and lactation	-if your blood sugars are not going down, but are going up (hyperglycemia)
Glimepiride* (Amaryl®)	1 to 2 mg once daily	8 mg once daily	With AM / First Meal		

*These drugs are available in generic, which means the generic alternatives are a cost savings to you!
**There are no fix doses for sulfonylureas, as the dosing depends on the individuals' glycemic control as determined by self monitoring of home blood glucose and the hemoglobin A1C, as well as, the health status of the individual.

Oral Antidiabetic Drug Class – Meglitinides (Insulin Secreting Agents)

Action: Helps the pancreas to secrete insulin

	Daily Dosing**		How To Take It	Take Note	Take Action
	Initial	Maximum			
				Expect to see lowering of blood glucose levels after the first dose.	May be helpful to test your blood glucose levels 2 hours after a meal, should be less than 180mg/dL
Benzoic Acid Derivative				These agents are taken before the meals to reduce the rise in glucose levels after a meal	Due to possible hypoglycemia, check your blood glucose levels regularly
Repaglinide (Prandin®)	0.5-2 mg 3-4 times a day	16 mg per day (Dosage range 0.5-4mg 4 times a day)	30 minutes to right before the meal	Hypoglycemia can occur in all patients, but mainly in patients: -older (> 65 years of age) and/or with liver or kidney problems -who have implemented an exercise program and/or reduced portion/caloric diet	If you skip a meal, skip the dose for that meal, this is very important Tell your provider:
D-Phenylalanine Derivative				Taking the medication and skipping the meal is a "no no". Skip dose if meal is skipped.	- if you are having more than 3 hypoglycemic reactions [< 70mg/dl per week (increase heart rate, sweating, hunger, lightheadedness)] Your dose may have to be adjusted
Nateglinide* (Starlix®)	60-120 mg three times daily	360 mg per day	30 minutes to right before the meal	Other side effects: weight gain, headache None of these agents are recommended in pregnancy and lactation	- if your blood sugars are not going down, but are going up (hyperglycemia)

**There are no fix doses for meglitinides, as the dosing depends on the individuals glycemic control as determined by self monitoring of home blood glucose and the hemoglobin A1C, as well as, the health status of the individual.

ORAL ANTIDIABETIC DRUG CLASS – THIAZOLIDINEDIONES (INSULIN SENSITIZERS)

	Daily Dosing**		How To Take It	TAKE NOTE	TAKE ACTION
	Initial	Maximum			
Action: Increases the sensitivity of the tissue (muscle, fat, liver) to insulin, increasing cell response to insulin				Expect to see maximum lowering of blood glucose levels after 2 months, but will see some lowering of blood glucose after 2 weeks	Due to possible hypoglycemia, and to make sure the medication is working check your blood glucose levels regularly.
				Hypoglycemia- can occur in all patients, mainly in patients:	Make sure your provider checks your liver with a blood test called liver function test before this therapy and periodically while you are on it. Have your provider share and discuss the results with you. The levels should not be 2.5 times the upper limit of normal.
Pioglitazone (Actos®)	15 - 30 mg once daily	45 mg once daily	With or without meals for both agents	- who are older(> 65 years of age) or have problems with their kidneys - who have implemented an exercise program and/or reduced portion/caloric diet - who are on other antidiabetic agents to lower glucose levels	Tell your provider: -if you are having more than 3 hypoglycemic reactions, [< 70mg/dL per week (increase heart rate, sweating, hunger, lightheadedness)] Your dose may have to be adjusted.
Rosiglitazone (Avandia®)	4 mg once daily or 2 mg twice daily	8 mg once daily or 4 mg twice daily		Must have a healthy liver to take this drug Other side effects: weight gain, fluid retention, swelling around the ankles None of these agents are recommended in pregnancy and lactation. **NOTE: These drugs may cause or worsen heart failure. If you have Class 3 or 4 Heart Failure, you should not take these drugs.**	- if you experience sudden increase in weight gain, swelling around the ankles, or shortness of breath -if you experience nausea, vomiting, dark urine, fatigue -if your blood sugars are not going down, but are going up (hyperglycemia)

**There are no fixed doses for Thiazolidinediones, as the dosing depends on the individuals' glycemic control as determined by self monitoring of home blood glucose and the hemoglobin A1C, as well as, the health status of the individual. Use of Rosiglitazone is severely restriced in the U.S. and other countries; Pioglitazone use has recently been restriced in France and Germany.

ORAL ANTIDIABETIC DRUG CLASS – THE BIGUANIDES (INSULIN SENSITIZERS)

Action: Increases the sensitivity of the tissue to insulin, to increase glucose uptake. Prevents the liver from making glucose.

	Daily Dosing**		How To Take It	TAKE NOTE	TAKE ACTION
	Initial	**Maximum**			
Metformin* (Glucophage®) (Immediate Release)	500 mg twice daily or 850 mg once daily	2000 mg daily dose divided 2-3 times daily	With Meals	-Usually reduction in glucose levels are seen at 1500 mg or at 3-4 weeks or earlier in some patients -Should not cause hypoglycemia when used alone, however, when combined with other antidiabetic agents, hypoglycemia can occur - May cause upset stomach and possible diarrhea, however this side effect does goes away with continued use - May also cause loss of appetite or metallic taste - You must have a healthy kidney and liver to take this drug	Monitor your blood glucose levels on a regular basis Be careful of hypoglycemia if on other antidiabetic agents When starting metformin titrating the dose up slowly helps to minimize any stomach upset or diarrhea. It helps to increase dose slowly by 500mg/week or as tolerated based on patient response blood test, ask your provider:
Metformin ER* (Fortamet®, Glucophage XR®) (Extended Release)	500 - 1000 once daily	2000 mg once daily (Glucophage XR) 2500 mg once daily (Fortamet)	With the evening meal	- Avoid in patients with renal failure or those who are predisposed to lactic acidosis, which is an increase in the acidity of your blood due to lack of blood oxygenation. Risk is increased with metformin use and in patients with acute heart attack, lung disease, chronic alcohol use, impaired kidneys or liver, radiological studies which require iodinated contrast dye, > 80 years of age with kidney dysfunction. - Should not be used in patients with congestive heart failure on therapy	Serum Creatinine, a measure of your kidney function should be done annually, for men it should be less than 1.5 mg/dl and women less than 1.4 mg/dl. If it is greater than these numbers, you should not be on metformin. Avoid excessive alcohol intake acutely or chronic Be familiar with the symptoms of lactic acidosis, and report to your provider
Metformin (Riomet®) (An Oral Solution 500mg/5ml)	500 mg twice daily	2550 mg daily dose divided 2-3 times daily	With Meals	-This drug can interfere with Vitamin B12 absorption but rarely causes anemia -Should not be used in pregnancy and/or lactation Good Effect - can cause modest weight loss the first couple of months after starting therapy	Breathing fast for no apparent reason, muscle aches, being sleepy or tired, stomach upset and diarrhea, which occurs after you have been stabilized on metformin.

*These drugs are available in generic, which means the generic alternatives are a cost savings to you!
**There are no fix doses for Biguanides, as the dosing depends on the individuals' glycemic control as determined by self monitoring of home blood glucose and the hemoglobin A1C, as well as, the health status of the individual.

ORAL ANTIDIABETIC DRUG CLASS – ALPHA-GLUCOSIDASE INHIBITORS

	Daily Dosing**		How To Take It	TAKE NOTE	TAKE ACTION
	Initial	Maximum			
Action: Changes the way your body absorbs sugars and starches after you eat, and prevents the sharp blood sugar spikes that occur, slowing the body's digestion of carbohydrates.				These agents are taken before the meals to reduce the rise in glucose levels after a meal Does not cause hypoglycemia on its on, but can when combined with insulin or other oral antidiabetic agents. Common side effects are diarrhea, upset stomach and gas. These effects diminish over time with continued use. May alter a blood test called liver function test Increase doses slowly to avoid GI effects. Should not use if you have trouble with digestion or stomach disorders Only use in pregnancy when benefits outweigh the risk. Do not use in breastfeeding women.	Monitor blood glucose levels regularly Due to possible hypoglycemia, check your blood glucose levels regularly. Ask your doctor to check your liver function test every 3 months for your first year on this drug and periodically thereafter, share the results with you and assure these are normal. Ask your doctor to check your kidneys with a blood test called Serum Creatinine, the result should be less than 2 mg/dL.
Acarbose* (Precose®)	25 mg three times daily	132 lbs (60 kg) 50 mg three times daily 132 lbs (60 kg) 100 mg three times daily	With the first bite of each main meal		
Miglitol * (Glyset®)	25 mg three times daily	100 mg three times daily	With the first bite of each main meal		

*There are no fixed doses for alpha glucosidase inhibitors as the dosing depends on the individuals' blood glucose control as determined by self-monitoring of blood glucose and the hemoglobin A1C as well as the health status of the individual

Oral Antidiabetic Drug Class – The Dipeptidyl Peptidase-IV (DPP-IV) Inhibitors

	Daily Dosing**		How To Take It	Take Note	Take Action
	Initial	Maximum			
Action: Prolongs the action of hormones called incretins that help the pancreas secrete insulin. It also stops the liver from making glucose.				When combined with other antidiabetic agents, hypoglycemia can occur.	Monitor your blood glucose levels on a regular basis.
Sitagliptin (Januvia®)	100 mg once daily	100 mg once daily	With or without Meals	Lower doses are recommended if you have kidney dysfunction. A dose of 25 mg per day is recommended if you are on dialysis.	Be careful of hypoglycemia if on other antidiabetic agents.
Saxagliptin (Onglyza®)	2.5 mg once daily	5 mg once dailyt	With or without Meals	Most common side effects are headache and upper respiratory infection.	Ask your doctor to check your liver function test every 3 months for your first year on this drug and periodically thereafter, share the results with you and assure these are normal.
Linagliptin (Tradjenta®)	5 mg once daily		With or without Meals	May use in pregnancy if benefits outweigh the risk. Studies have not been done in pregnant women, however it did not result in problems with pregnant rats.	You should not take these drugs if you have severe liver problems.
Alogliptin (Not Known as yet)	25 mg once daily			May use in breast feeding with caution. Drug is excreted in breast milk with rats. Studies have not been done in women	Ask your doctor to check your kidneys with a blood test called Serum Creatinine, the result should be less than 2 mg/dl

**There are no fix doses for DPP-IV Inhibitors, as the dosing depends on the individuals glycemic control as determined by self monitoring of home blood glucose and the hemoglobin A1C, as well as, the health status of the individual.

ORAL ANTIDIABETIC DRUG CLASS – CENTRALLY ACTING DOPAMINE AGONIST BROMOCRIPTINE* (CYCLOSET)

Action: Decreases postprandial plasma glucose levels without increasing plasma insulin concentrations in patients with type 2 diabetes

	Daily Dosing**		How To Take It	Take Note	Take Action
	Initial	Maximum			
Bromocriptine* (Cycloset®)	0.8 mg (1 tablet) once daily	4.8 mg (6 tablets) once daily	Take orally in the morning, within two hours after waking, with food	These drug is taken orally in the morning, within 2 hours after waking	Monitor blood glucose levels regularly
				Take with food to reduce the risk of nausea	Due to possible hypoglycemia, check your blood glucose levels regularly.
				Common side effects are fatigue, nausea, vomiting, dizziness and headache	Ask your doctor to check your liver function test every 3 months for your first year on this drug and periodically thereafter, share the results with you and assure you that these are normal.
				May alter a blood test called liver function test	
				May use in pregnancy only if benefits outweigh the risk. Do **NOT** use in breastfeeding women.	Ask your doctor to check your kidneys with a blood test called Serum Creatinine; the result should be less than 2 mg/dL.

*There are no fixed doses for Bromocriptine, as the dosing depends on the individuals' blood glucose control as determined by self-monitoring of blood glucose and the hemoglobin A1C as well as the health status of the individual

Injectable Antidiabetic Drug Class Amylin Analog - Pramlintide (Symlin®)(Solution for Injection)

	Daily Dosing				
	Initial	Maximum	How To Take It	Take Note	Take Action
Action: Reduces glucose levels by reducing the amount of glucose the liver makes. Slows the emptying of the stomach.				Indicated for Type 1 and Type 2 patients who are on mealtime insulin and have suboptimal glucose control	Monitor your blood glucose levels on a regular basis
				Hypoglycemia can occur up to 3 hours after a dose. Alcohol can intensify the hypoglycemia	When you first start this drug, or the dose is increased, do not drive or operate heavy machinery up to 3 hours after dose due to possible hypoglycemia
Type 1 Diabetics Pramlintide (Symlin®)	15 mcg/ meal	30-60 mcg/meal	Take/give at mealtimes, immediately prior to each <u>major meal</u>	Does not replace your pre-mealtime insulin, but dose of pre-mealtime insulin can be reduced. Do not mix insulin with pramlintide in the same syringe.	
			Major meal (250 calories or equal to or 30 grams of carbohydrate). Given by subcutaneous injection: in the thigh or abdomen.	Allow the solution to reach room temperature before administering to reduce injection site reactions.	Take other oral drugs one hour before taking pramlintide, or 2 hours after, to prevent pramlintide from slowing their absorption.
			<u>DO NOT ADMINISTER IN THE ARM.</u> Rotate injection sites frequently.	Type 2 patients, in addition to insulin can take metformin or a sulfonylurea	
Type 2 Diabetics Pramlintide* (Symlin®)	60 mcg/ meal	120 mcg/meal	Inject 2 inches away from the insulin injection site	Nausea is most common side effect but may diminish over time with continue use. Causes a feeling of fullness and therefore may reduce appetite and cause weight loss. Because pramlintide slows gastric emptying, it can slow the absorption of other drugs taken orally.	Initially when combined with insulin, (rapid, regular, or fixed with rapid or regular) the insulin dose must be reduced <u>by 50%</u> to prevent hypoglycemia.
				May use in pregnancy if benefits outweigh the risk. May use in breast feeding with caution	

*There are no fix doses for pramlintide, as the dosing depends on the incivduals glycemic control as determined by self monitoring of home blood glucose and the hemoglobin A1C, as well as, the health status of the individual

INJECTABLE ANTIDIABETIC DRUG CLASS (TYPE 2 DIABETICS ONLY) LIRAGLUTIDE (VICTOZA®)

	Initial	Maximum	How To Take It	Take Note	Take Action
Action: Reduces glucose levels by reducing the amount of glucose the liver makes, increase insulin secretion. Slows the emptying of the stomach.				When combined with other antidiabetic agents, hypoglycemia can occur. Because liraglutide slows gastric emptying, it can slow the absorption of other drugs taken orally. Most common side effects are headache, nausea and diarrhea.	Monitor your blood glucose levels on a regular basis Be careful of hypoglycemia (shakiness, sweating, drowsiness, dizziness, fast heartbeat, hunger) if on other antidiabetic agents
Liraglutide (Victoza®) (A injectable pen device)	0.6 mg daily	1.8 mg daily	Can be taken with or without food. Inject one time per day at any time of the day. Inject under the skin in the abdomen thigh or upper arm as instructed.	You should not use this drug if you have gallstones, pancreatitis, high lipids in your blood and if you drink alcohol or have done so in the past. The risks for use in pregnancy and breastfeeding are not known. If you take too much Victoza call your doctor right away. Do not share pens with anyone even though the needle is changed. There is risk of contracting an infection if pens are shared. Store the pens in the refrigerator prior to first use. Do not freeze. After first use the pen may be stored for 30 days at controlled room temperature. Do not keep in excessive heat and sunlight. Remove and discard the needle after each use. Store the pen in the refrigerator without a needle attached. Pen needles are not included and need to be purchased separately.	Take other oral drugs one hour before taking liraglutide, to prevent the slowing of absorption of other drugs. Report immediately to your doctor any pain in your stomach area that is severe and will not go away.

Injectable Antidiabetic Drug Class
Incretin Mimetics (Type 2 Diabetics Only)
Exenatide (Byetta®)

	Initial	Maximum	How To Take It	Take Note	Take Action
Action: Reduces glucose levels by reducing the amount of glucose the liver makes, increase insulin secretion. Slows the emptying of the stomach.					
Exenatide (Byetta®) (A injectable pen device)	5 mcg/dose twice daily	10 mcg/dose twice daily	Take within 60 minutes prior to morning and evening meal or prior to the 2 main meals of the day approximately 6 hours apart Given by subcutaneous injection: in the thigh, abdomen, or upper arm Can be added to a sulfonylurea or metformin	When combined with other antidiabetic agents, hypoglycemia can occur. Hypoglycemia more common when used with a sulfonylurea than with metformin. Sulfonylurea dose may have to be lowered. Because exenatide slows gastric emptying, it can slow the absorption of other drugs taken orally. If you miss a dose before a meal, do not take after a meal, just take the next scheduled dose Causes a feeling of fullness and therefore may reduce appetite and cause weight loss. Most common side effects are diarrhea, nausea, vomiting. You should not use this drug if you have gallstones, pancreatitis, high lipids in your blood and if you drink alcohol or have done so in the past.	Monitor your blood glucose levels on a regular basis Be careful of hypoglycemia if on other antidiabetic agents Take other oral drugs one hour before taking exenatide, to prevent exenatide from slowing their absorption. Report to your doctor any pain in your stomach area that is severe and will not go away. You should tell your doctor if you have

ORAL ANTIDIABETIC COMBINATION AGENTS	TAKE NOTE	TAKE ACTION
Sulfonylurea + Metformin	These agents should be initiated after you have been on one of the agents alone, but still need additional glucose lowering or you have been stabilized on both agents.	Check blood glucose levels regularly.
Glyburide/metformin* (Glucovance®)		Notify your provider if you have greater than 3 low blood sugar reactions (hypoglycemia) in one week.
Glipizide/metformin* (Metaglip®)	If you never have been on either agent alone or together, it is not recommended to start two new agents at once because of the increased risk of hypoglycemia and may not be able to tell the cause of an allergic reaction.	
Thiazolidinedione + Sulfonylurea		
Pioglitazone/glimepiride (Duetact®)	The advantage of these agents is one pill contains two medications. Any increase in dose is dependent on which drug is being adjusted.	
Rosiglitazone/glimepiride (Avandaryl®)		
Thiazolidinedione + Metformin	Please refer to previous drug charts to for additional information on each individual agent.	
Rosiglitazone/metformin (Avandamet®)		
Pioglitazone/metformin (ActoPlus Met®)		
Metformin + DPP IV Inhibitor		
Sitagliptin/ Metformin (Janumet®)		
Saxagliptin/Metformin (Kombiglyze®)		
Meglitinide + Metformin		
Repaglinide /Metformin (PrandiMet®)		

*Only Glucovance® and Metaglip® combinations are available in generic. Use of Rosiglitazone is severely restriced in the U.S. and other countries; Pioglitazone use has recently been restriced in France and Germany..

Future Diabetes Drugs

Dapaglifolozin

A novel approach to treating diabetes is the reduction of high blood glucose levels by removing excess glucose in the urine. Dapaglifolozin is a sodium glucose co-transporter (SGLT2) inhibitor. This drug inhibits SGLT2, allowing the kidney to reabsorb less glucose and therefore excrete excess glucose in the urine lowering the concentration of glucose in the urine thus lowering glucose levels in the blood. This reduction in blood glucose is not associated with hypoglycemia This future drug can be used as monotherapy or as add-on to metformin for patients who are diagnosed with type 2 diabetes. Reducing hyperglycemia is a challenge in the management of diabetes to avoid acute symptoms and especially to reduce the complications that are associated with diabetes. Dapaglifolozin potentially reduces hyperglycemia and also causes weight loss.

Bydureon

Bydureon is an injectable once weekly form of Exenatide Byetta®. It mimics the hormone incretin, which is released after a meal and slows digestion. It is a long acting form of the drug easier and more convenient to use, because it is used once weekly compared to twice daily. Bydureon lowers fasting glucose levels, and helps with weight loss. It also helps to lower HbA1c levels. Chemically, it is very similar to glucagon which is something your body naturally secrets after eating. This chemical helps to digest food and let the body know that it has received food. The side effects nausea, diarrhea and vomiting are similar to Byetta®. Bydureon is recommended for use in patients with type 2 diabetes who are be already using another oral antidiabetic drug.

Test Your Knowledge

Oral Antidiabetic Medications

1. If you have Type 1 diabetes you will need to use insulin for the rest of your life to control your blood sugar. With Type 2 diabetes your blood sugar can be adequately controlled with a combination of diet, exercise and oral medications.

   TRUE   FALSE

2. The agents that control after meal spikes in blood glucose (postprandial hyperglycemia(include:

   a) Alpha glucosidase inhibitors
   b) Fast acting insulin analogs
   c) Thiazolidinediones

   1) a,b,c
   2) a,c
   3) c only
   4) all of the above

3. The two classes of oral medications that do not cause weight gain are

   a) Alpha Glucosidase inhibitors
   b) Sulfonylureas
   c) Biguanides
   d) Meglitinides

   1) a,c
   2) b,c
   3) b,d
   4) c,d

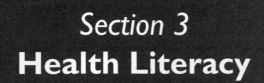

Section 3
Health Literacy

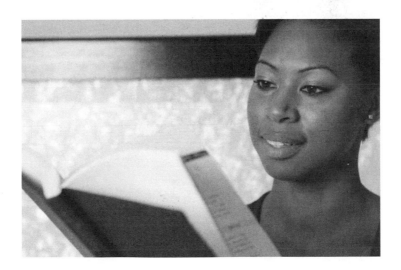

Health Literacy

In **Health Literacy: A Prescription to End Confusion**, the Institute of Medicine reports that ninety (90) million people in the United States, nearly half the population, have difficulty understanding and using health information. As a result, many patients often do not take their medications as prescribed, miss follow-up appointments with their health care provider and do not understand medication instructions like "take on an empty stomach."

The people most affected by health literacy are the medically underserved, vulnerable populations.

These tend to be the:

- Elderly (age 65+) - Two thirds of U.S. adults age 60 and over have inadequate or marginal literacy skills, and 81% of patients age 60 and older at a public hospital could not read or understand basic materials such as prescription labels
- Minority populations (African American, Latinos, Native Americans, Asians and Hawaiian Islanders)
- Immigrant populations
- Low income - Approximately half of Medicare/Medicaid recipients read below the fifth-grade level
- People with chronic mental and/or physical health conditions

Reasons for limited literacy skills include:

- Lack of educational opportunity - people with a high school education or lower
- Learning disabilities
- Cognitive declines in older adults

Use it or lose it - Reading abilities are typically three to five grade levels below the last year of school completed. Therefore, people with a high school diploma typically read at a seventh or eighth grade reading level.

The relationship between literacy and health is complex. Literacy impacts health knowledge, health status, and access to health services. Health status is influenced by several related socioeconomic factors. Literacy impacts income level, occupation, education, housing, and access to medical care. The poor and illiterate are more likely to work under hazardous conditions or be exposed to environmental toxins.

Health literacy includes the ability to understand instructions on prescription drug bottles, appointment slips, medical education brochures, doctor's directions and consent forms, and the ability to negotiate complex health care systems. Health literacy is not simply the ability to read. It requires a complex group of reading, listening, analytical, and decision-making skills, and the ability to apply these skills to health situations. In this chapter we are going to review two important aspects of health literacy, medication compliance and how to talk with your healthcare provider.

Medication Adherence

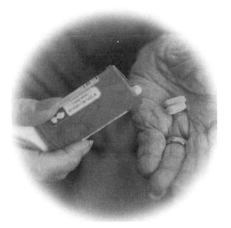

Two-thirds of all Americans fail to take any or all of their prescription medications. Almost 29% of Americans stop taking their medications before they run out. Twelve percent (12%) of Americans do not take their medications as prescribed, after they buy the prescription.

Here are some helpful hints to improve your compliance with your medication regimen.

- Always get your medication filled on time and from the same pharmacy so that they can have a complete record of your medication history.
- Don't stop taking a prescribed medication because your symptoms have gone away or you feel better. Diabetes and high blood pressure are chronic conditions that will require long-term treatment.
- Always check with your health care provider before you stop taking a medication.
- If you are experiencing side effects from your medications, mention it to your health care provider so that he/she can change or modify your medication regimen.
- If you miss taking a medication, do not double up.
- If you see multiple physicians, make sure they all know what medicines you are taking.
- Keep a written record of medications that you are taking. Write down the names, strengths and directions for use. Keep this record with you at all times.
- Do not share or borrow medications from anyone else.
- Store your medications in a cool, dry place. Always check the expiration date to make sure your medications are not expired.
- If you have diabetes and/or high blood pressure, check with your pharmacist before you buy over-the-counter medications. Some of these medications may increase your blood pressure and blood sugar.

Tips on How to Talk with Your Health Care Provider

In order to have a successful encounter with your healthcare provider you need to ask yourself the following questions.

- Do you feel comfortable talking with your healthcare provider (clinician)?
- Does he or she do all the talking while you do all the listening?
- Are you afraid to ask questions because you are embarrassed or afraid of looking dumb?
- Do you leave the office feeling like you just sat through a foreign language class?

Improving your relationship with your health care provider is based on how well you communicate with each other. Good communication can improve your care and improve your relationship with your healthcare team. A good relationship — where you and your clinician share information and work together to make the best decisions about your health — will result in the best care. You'll also feel more confident in your clinician and the quality of care you're getting.

Here are some ways to make talking to your health care team more effective.

Be Prepared

Healthcare providers are busy people and their offices are often full of activity, like ringing telephones and crowded waiting rooms. When you actually see your doctor, your visit probably won't last more than 10 - 15 minutes.

The best way to make the most of your limited time is to come to your appointment prepared:

Write down all the questions you have for the doctor in advance and bring a pen and paper to jot down answers and take notes.

Make and bring a list of symptoms if you're not feeling well. You might want to research your condition at the library or on the internet if you're visiting your doctor for a specific problem or illness. Learning some related medical terms and common treatments will make it easier to follow what the doctor is telling you.

Bring a list of all the medicines you take. Write down the doses and how often you take them. Include vitamins, other supplements, and over-the- counter medicines you take on a regular basis.

Arrive early enough to fill out forms.

Have your insurance card ready and bring your medical records or have them sent in advance if you're seeing the doctor for the first time. Also bring your health care advance directive, which outlines instructions about your care if you become unable to speak for yourself. Go over it with your doctor so that your wishes are clear. Make sure you have designated someone in your family or a close friend (with a medical background) to have your durable power of attorney for health care. Discuss your wishes for advance life support with that person so that they know your wishes in case you are unable to speak for yourself.

Here are some questions you should come prepared to ask your clinician. You can add to the list as you come up with more questions.

Problem

- What is wrong with me? How do you know?
- What do you think caused this problem?
- Will my problem go away or is it a chronic condition that can be controlled by not CURED?

Tests Used in My Diagnosis

- Must I have tests? Will I have to take the tests again?

- What tests do I need and why?
- What do the tests involve?
- How do I prepare for the tests?
- When will I know the test results?
- Will my insurance cover the cost of the tests?

Treatment

- What are my different treatment choices?
- What are the benefits and risks of each treatment?
- What are the common side effects of the medications you are prescribing for me to take?
- How effective is each treatment?
- Which treatment have you found to work in most patients?
- What do I do if the treatment fails?

Medication

- What kind of medication(s) must I take for my condition? For how long will I need to take the medication?
- What does the medication do? Will there be any side effects?
- What should I do if I have side effects?
- Can I take a generic version of the drug?
- Will the medicine interact with any I am already taking?
- Should I avoid any kind of food or activity while taking this medicine?

Medical Consultation

- Do I need to see a specialist?
- Should I get a second opinion?

Speak Up

Don't be put off by big words or a health care provider's impatient manner. If you don't understand what the doctor is telling you, ask him or her to explain it again. Using different words, or drawing or showing you a picture can help. Don't leave the office without understanding everything the clinician has told you.

If there are issues you want to discuss that the clinician doesn't mention, raise them yourself. Clinicians often are so focused on making sick people better — or so rushed — they forget to talk about important health matters like diet and weight, exercise, stress, sleep, tobacco and alcohol use, sexual practices, vaccines, and tests to find diseases. Find out what tests you might need for your age, such as a mammogram, prostate exam or colonoscopy, and ask your doctor about getting them.

Don't be embarrassed or ashamed to bring up sensitive topics. Do not withhold information. Speaking up also means telling your doctor everything you know about your body and health, including all your symptoms and problems. The more information you share, the better the clinician will be able to figure out what's wrong and how to treat you. Don't make the clinician guess. Be sure to mention any and all medicines, vitamins, and herbs you are taking, and anyone else you are seeing about your health, physical and mental well being.

Bring a Family Member or Friend with You to Your Appointment

Sometimes, people like to bring a friend or family member to a medical appointment for moral support. A companion also could help you relax, remind you of questions you forgot to ask, and help you remember what the doctor said. If you need personal time with the clinician, the person can sit in the waiting room. Having someone join you is especially helpful if you feel too ill to get around easily on your own.

Follow Up

If you feel nervous, rushed, or just plain overwhelmed, you might forget to ask a question, even if you wrote it down. If this happens, or if you think of a new question, call the office right away. Be patient but firm if you want to speak directly with the clinician, who might not be able to take your call at that moment. If the clinician wants you to come back for a follow up visit, be sure to set and keep the appointment.

Building a successful partnership with your health care provider takes time and effort. It's not uncommon to have a frustrating medical visit now and then. But overall, your relationship with your clinician should be positive and comfortable. You should have confidence and trust in his or her medical ability and judgment.

In the end, the most important aspect of your relationship with your healthcare provider is **TRUST**. You must trust your health care provider and feel they are able to help you improve your overall health. If you feel that you are not getting the care that you deserve you may want to consider changing your health care provider.

What important healthcare documents should I request and keep in my possession?

It is important that you have access to your medical information. When you go to your doctor, request a copy of your medical record. If you doctor is using Electronic Health Records (EHR) asked to be allowed computer access to your medical record. Electronic Health Records will allow you to have up to date information on your medical condition, laboratory and diagnostic tests. You can also share information with your doctor and be able to ask questions and be in constant contact with your doctor and the healthcare team. You can actually put your medical information into a Personalized Health Record (PHR) that is available either through your doctor's office or on the internet. Having a PHR will help you keep your medical and health information current and is very handy if you travel to other parts of the world since it is available on the internet in a SECURE platform. It is also important that you have your doctor write a permission slip for you to obtain your pharmacy and laboratory records. You need to keep an up to date records of your most recent laboratory tests and a list of ALL YOUR MEDICATIONS both prescription and over the counter.

Test Your Knowledge

Health Literacy

1. The Institute of Medicine reports that 90 million people in the United States have difficulty understanding and using health information.

   TRUE   FALSE

2. The people most affected by health literacy are

   a) Minority populations and immigrants
   b) Middle income patients
   c) Low income patients and those with chronic mental illness
   d) Adolescent patients

   1) a,b,c.   2) b,d   3) a,c   4) all of the above

3. Two-thirds (2/3) of all Americans fail to take any or all of their prescription medications.

   TRUE   FALSE

4. Reasons for limited literacy include learning disabilities and the lack of educational opportunity

   TRUE   FALSE

5. The most important requirement in building a relationship with your healthcare provider is:

   a) Trust
   b) Location of the medical office
   c) A friendly office staff
   d) Access to health information

   1) a   2) b   3) c   4) d

Section 4
Diabetes Complications

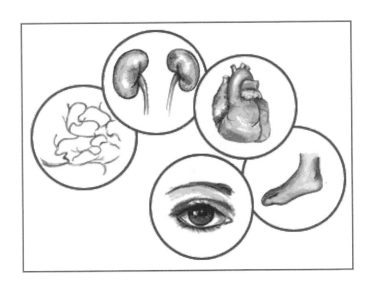

Complications of Diabetes

Are there other things I need to know about my diabetes?

You should know what other problems might happen due to your diabetes. These things may not happen to everyone. You are more likely than other people without diabetes to have problems with your eyes, kidneys and feet, in addition to strokes (brain attacks) and heart attacks. You are also more likely to get infections and have sexual problems. These complications mentioned above are generally due to high glucose levels in the blood which cause damage to nerves, small and large blood vessels, and reduced ability of your body to fight off infections.

What problems occur when my small blood vessels are damaged?

Diabetes can damage the small blood vessels in your eyes and kidneys. When your blood sugar is high and remains high for long periods of time these small blood vessels become damaged, swollen and leaky.

Blindness can occur as a result of the disease process occurring in the eyes, called **retinopathy**, a condition consisting of damage to the retina (the back of the eye). Although it occurs very slowly, eye damage is a very serious complication.

In addition, damage to the small blood vessels in the kidney results in **nephropathy**, which is the medical term for kidney damage. The kidneys filter out the waste in the blood and pass them into the urine. High blood glucose and high blood pressure damage the blood vessels and the filtering ability of the kidneys. Damage to the filtering system of the kidney causes waste products to stay in the blood. When the kidneys are damaged, things such as protein leave the blood and spill into the urine. If damage continues, the kidneys will stop working.

Why do I need to take care of my eyes and my kidneys?

A simple eye exam tells the health care provider if you have retinopathy and how severe it is. People with Type 1 diabetes for over 5 years should have an eye exam every year. People with Type 2 diabetes should have their eyes checked when they find out they have diabetes and every year thereafter. Better control of blood glucose helps control eye problems. If you have had diabetes for a long time, these eye problems will probably not go away. One of the first signs that you may notice is that your vision is blurry. This happens because the high blood glucose causes nerve damage in the eyes. If you notice blurry vision, you should tell your health care provider. Your health care provider may send you to a special doctor (ophthalmologist) who will check your eyes very closely. You are more likely to get other eye diseases such as glaucoma and cataracts. Once again, if your health care provider finds eye disease early enough, eye damage is less likely.

It is very important for you to tell your health care provider if you are having any problems with your eyes or if you notice any changes in how your eyes look. Always have your eyes checked at least once a year.

Your health care provider can check for protein in the urine (proteinuria). The first sign of kidney disease is called microalbuminura (small amounts of protein in the urine), which can be reversible if blood glucose levels are improved. The test that identifies protein in the urine is called the spot urine collection test. A normal result is less than 30 ug/mg of creatinine. The presence of consistent high blood pressure worsens proteinuria in people with diabetes. Protein in urine has been shown to predict the possibility of dying early from diabetes, due to kidney disease. It is important that you check how well your kidneys are functioning at least twice a year when you see your health care provider.

What about nerve damage and sexual problems?

Your nerves are like telephone or electrical lines that help different parts of your body talk to each other. Diabetes quite often damages your nerves. **Neuropathy** is the medical term for nerve damage. High blood glucose is often the cause of this damage. When this occurs, the nerves do not send out their signals as well as before. Some of the signs of nerve damage in the feet and legs include numbness, tingling ("pins and needles sensation"), burning, and aching. Sometimes the damage is so serious that injuries happen to the feet and legs and the patient does not know these injuries have happened. Damage to the nerves puts you at risk for foot injury, infection and amputation.

Diabetes can cause sexual problems through nerve damage. Men may be less likely to get and/or keep an erection. Women may be less likely to have an orgasm. These problems can usually be treated through aggressive blood glucose control.

What problems occur when my large blood vessels are damaged?

Diabetes can damage the large blood vessels in your arms, legs, and around the heart. The vessels become stiff and hard and allow the trapping of cholesterol. Trapping of enough cholesterol leads to blockage of these large blood vessels and makes your heart work harder to pump the blood. Overworking your heart too long leads to strokes, heart attacks and high blood pressure. Also, trapped cholesterol can cause poor circulation in your arms and legs. Heart disease and stroke account for 65 percent of deaths in people with diabetes. The death rate for people with diabetes is 2-5 times higher than people without diabetes. The risk of stroke is 2-4 times higher and the risk of death from stroke is 2 times higher among people with diabetes.

Why do I sometimes have trouble fighting off infections?

Small blood vessel and nerve damage can make infections in people with diabetes difficult to treat. Poor blood flow and high blood glucose slow down the body's infection fighting team, the white blood cells. High glucose levels are a breeding ground for bacteria. Nerve damage prevents you from knowing when you injure yourself. A cut or scrape may turn into a serious infection if it is not treated quickly. People with prediabetes or diabetes may also experience frequent urinary tract or vaginal infections due to high glucose levels.

The best way to treat all of these conditions (damage to blood vessels, nerves, sexual function, and frequent infections) is to keep close control over your blood glucose. Through careful monitoring and medication usage, you can keep these problems to a minimum. By controlling high blood pressure, decreasing blood cholesterol, giving up smoking, and regular eye, kidney and foot exams, you may lessen the risks.

Are there certain ethnic groups at increased risk of diabetes complications?

Compared with white Americans, African Americans experience higher rates of diabetes complications such as eye disease, kidney failure and amputations. They also experience greater disability from these complications. Some factors that influence the frequency of these complications such as high blood glucose levels, abnormal blood lipids, high blood pressure and cigarette smoking, can be influenced by proper diabetes management.

Eye Disease leading to Blindness

African Americans are almost 40- 50 percent as likely to develop diabetic retinopathy as Caucasians according to the NHANES III data. The reason that retinopathy occurs more frequently in African Americans has to do with the higher rate of hypertension.

Kidney Failure leading to End Stage Renal Disease (ESRD) and Dialysis

African Americans are 2.6 to 5.6 times as likely to suffer from kidney disease. African Americans with diabetes, experience kidney failure, also called end stage renal disease (ESRD), about four times more often than other patients with diabetes. Diabetes related kidney failure accounts for 43% of the new cases of End State Renal Disease (ESRD). More than 4,000 new cases of End Stage Renal Disease (ESRD) occur each year.

Amputations

African Americans are 2.7 times as likely to suffer from lower-limb amputations. Amputation rates are 1.4 to 2.7 times higher in men than women with diabetes. Based on a study from Northwestern University's Feinburg School of Medicine, African Americans had five times higher rate of lower limb amputation than Caucasians in the Chicago area. African American patients have skin ulcers and gangrene that if left untreated or not treated with the latest wound care advances. It is important that you care for your skin and feet so that you do not have problems later in life.

Heart Disease

African American adults are more likely to be diagnosed with coronary heart disease, and they are more likely to die from heart disease. Although African American adults are 40% more likely to have high blood pressure, they are 10% less likely than their non-Hispanic White counterparts to have their blood pressure under control.

- In 2007, African American men were 30% more likely to die from heart disease, as compared to non-Hispanic white men.

- African Americans are 1.5 times as likely as non-Hispanic whites to have high blood pressure.

Excess Deaths in African Americans

Diabetes was an uncommon cause of death among African Americans at the turn of the century. By 1994, however, death certificates listed diabetes as the seventh leading cause of death for African Americans. For those 45 years or older, it was the fifth leading cause of death. In every age group and for both men and women, death rates for African Americans with diabetes are higher than for whites with diabetes. Death rates for people with diabetes are higher for African Americans than for whites. A national survey conducted from 1971-1993, noted that the overall mortality rate of African American men was 20% higher for African American men and 40% higher for African American women, compared with their white counterparts.

Why do I sometimes have trouble fighting off infections?

Small blood vessel and nerve damage can make infections in people with diabetes difficult to treat. Poor blood flow and high blood glucose slow down the body's infection fighting team, the white blood cells. High glucose levels are a breeding ground for bacteria. Nerve damage prevents you from knowing when you injure yourself. A cut or scrape may turn into a serious infection if it is not treated quickly. People with diabetes or prediabetes may also experience frequent urinary tract or vaginal infections due to high glucose levels.

The best way to treat all of these conditions (damage to blood vessels, nerves, sexual function, and frequent infections) is to keep close control over your blood glucose. Through careful monitoring and medication usage, you can keep these problems to a minimum. By controlling high blood pressure, decreasing blood cholesterol, giving up smoking, and regular eye, kidney and foot exams, you may lessen the risks.

Test Your Knowledge
Diabetes Complications

1. The complications of diabetes can occur due to damage to the small blood vessels and large blood vessels. Damage to the small blood vessels can cause:

   a) eye problems (retinopathy)
   b) kidney problems (nephropathy)
   c) nerve problems (neuropathy)
   d) strokes/heart attacks

   1) a,b,c
   2) a,c
   3) b,d
   4) all of the above

2. Your health care provider should check for protein in your urine (microalbumin) on a regular basis to make sure that you do not have kidney disease.
   TRUE   FALSE

3. In order to prevent blindness and kidney failure you should

   a) have your eyes checked by an ophthalmologist yearly
   b) control your blood sugar
   c) control your blood pressure

   1) a,b,c
   2) a,c
   3) c only

4. Often, people with diabetes have trouble fighting off infections.

   TRUE   FALSE

High Blood Pressure

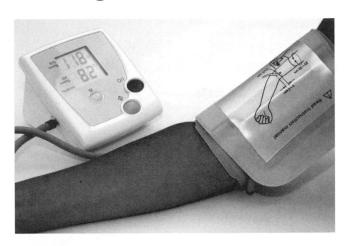

Who has high blood pressure?

It is estimated that nearly 74.5 million Americans (age 20 and older) have high blood pressure. One in three U.S. adults have high blood pressure. Of those people with high blood pressure, 77.6 percent do not know they have it. High blood pressure or "hypertension," as it is also known, is one of the most dangerous diseases in our country. High blood pressure killed approximately 54,186 Americans in 2004 and contributed to the death of 277,000. If left untreated, it can increase the risk of heart attacks, strokes and heart failure.

In most cases, we don't know what causes high blood pressure. But the good news is that it can be treated, and there are things that you can do to reduce your chances of getting high blood pressure.

What is blood pressure and why is it harmful?

Arteries carry blood from the heart to all parts of the body. The force of blood pushing against the walls of the arteries is blood pressure. Each time the heart beats, it pumps blood into the arteries. Blood pressure is highest when the heart contracts and is pumping blood; this is called the systolic pressure. Between beats, when the heart is at rest, the blood pressure falls; this is the diastolic pressure.

High blood pressure causes the blood vessels to get stiff and narrow. This makes the heart work harder to get the blood through your vessels. High blood pressure can also weaken the lining of the arteries and veins so that it is more susceptible to cholesterol deposits. This narrowing of the blood vessels throughout the body can lead to problems with the heart, kidneys, brain and eyes.

Measuring your blood pressure

A blood pressure measurement is given as two numbers. When written, for example, the number might be 120/80; this blood pressure, when spoken, is "120 over 80." The higher (top) number (120) is the systolic pressure, while the lower (bottom) number (80) is the diastolic pressure. These numbers are measurements of millimeters (mm) of mercury (Hg). A blood pressure reading of less than 120/80 mm Hg for adults is considered normal, (see Table 19 at the end of this section). High blood pressure is grouped by stages, and the higher the number, the more serious the problem.

The goal blood pressure for patients with hypertension and no other conditions is less than 140/90 mmHg. However, if a patient has diabetes or kidney disease the blood pressure goal is less than 130/80 mmHg. It has been proposed that the target blood pressure for African Americans is 120/80 mmHg. Persons with diabetes require the lowest levels of blood pressure in order to achieve protection from heart attacks, and damage to the kidneys. It is most important that blood pressure is aggressively treated in people with diabetes.

Are there certain ethnic groups at increased risk?

African Americans in the United States have the highest rate of hypertension in the world. Thirty percent (30%) of all deaths in African American men and 20% of all deaths in African American women are due to high blood pressure. African Americans are four times more likely to have hypertension than Caucasians. (See Figure 3 at the end of this section). Hypertension runs in families. If you have a family history of hypertension make sure that everyone in your immediate and extended family gets his or her blood pressure checked. The hypertension that you see in African Americans is more severe and occurs at an earlier age. According to the latest statistics from the American Heart Association (www.heart.org), hypertension was the primary or contributing cause of death in 319,000 people in the year 2005. 12,765 African Americans died from high blood pressure in 2005. High blood pressure causes damage to the heart and blood vessels that can lead to heart disease and stroke. African Americans die 1.5 times more frequently from heart disease and 1.8 times more frequently from strokes than Caucasians. Twenty six percent (26%) of all new cases of kidney failure each year are due to high blood pressure. There are a number of factors that contribute to the high blood pressure seen in African Americans:

- Eating a diet high in salt content.
- Not eating enough potassium and calcium.
- Being overweight.
- A sedentary lifestyle.
- Fewer physician visits.
- Not taking their medications as prescribed.
- Genetic factors.

What are the signs of high blood pressure?

You could have high blood pressure and not even know it—that's why it's often called the "silent killer." Approximately 28% of people with high blood pressure don't know they have it. There are usually no warning signs for high blood pressure. Many people don't find out they have high blood pressure until they have trouble with their heart, brain or kidneys.

Some of the symptoms of high blood pressure include:

- Dizziness
- Headache
- Blurred vision
- Rapid heart beat

What is the treatment of high blood pressure?

When you find out that you have high blood pressure, it is important that you understand that it can be controlled but not cured. You must make the decision to take control of your condition and make the changes in your lifestyle that will be necessary to control your blood pressure. It is not going to be easy, but there are a few simple steps that you can take.

Stop smoking—Even 1-3 cigarettes per day can increase your risk for heart attacks and strokes, so you must quit altogether.

Limit your alcohol intake—No more than one glass of alcohol per day for women and two drinks per day for men. One drink is 12 oz. of beer, 5 oz. wine and 1.5 oz. of 80-proof liquor.

Cut down on salt—The average American diet contains 25 grams of sodium. If you have high blood pressure, you should eat no more than 2.4 grams (2400 milligrams) of sodium per day. Avoid foods that are high in salt (potato chips, deli meats, canned soups). Use herbs and spices to season your food instead of seasoning salt. Read the nutrition labels of the foods that you eat and count every mg of sodium.

Lose weight— Currently 66% of the U.S. population is overweight and 34% are obese. African Americans have more obesity than Caucasians. We are now seeing an epidemic of obesity in our children, especially teenagers. Being overweight can place an increased burden on the heart and can make your hypertension worse. It is important that we begin taking off the excess weight by combining regularexercise with a well-balanced, low-fat diet.

What type of medications do you use to treat high blood pressure?

Currently there are multiple medications that can be used to treat high blood pressure. In order to achieve a goal blood pressure of 140/90 mmHg, many people may require 2-3 different medications taken at the same time. Keep in mind; the goal blood pressure for people with diabetes is less than 130/80 mmHg. The different classes of medications have specific mechanisms of action. Compaired to whites, most African Americans will require a diuretic (water pill) to reach their goal blood pressure. On the following pages, there are tables which provide some information regarding some of the common medications used in the treatment of high blood pressure. It is important that you take your medications as prescribed.

Table 19. Categories for Blood Pressure Levels in Adults*

CATEGORY	SYSTOLIC	DIASTOLIC
Normal	<120	and <80
Prehypertension	120 - 139	Or 80 - 89
Stage 1 Hypertension	140 - 159	Or 90 - 99
Stage 2 Hypertension	> or = 160	> or = 100

*For those not taking medicine for high blood pressure and not having a short-term serious illness. These categories are from the National High Blood Pressure Education Program (< means less than; > means greater than or equal to) +Normal Blood Pressure with respect to cardiovascular risk is below 120/80 mmHg. However, unusually low readings should be evaluated for clinical significance.

Commonly Used High Blood Pressure Medications

NAME OF MEDICATION	HOW THEY WORK TO LOWER YOUR BLOOD PRESSURE	POSSIBLE SIDE EFFECTS	COMMENTS
Diuretics ("water pills")			
Thiazide Diuretics Chlorthalidone* (Hygroton®) Hydrochlorothiazide* (Esidrix®) metolazone (Zaroxylyn®) Indapamide* (Lozo®)	Decrease blood pressure by eliminating excess fluid and salt (sodium)	Frequent urination, may decrease potassium levels (Note: potassium is a chemical in the body that helps to regulate your heart)	Certain foods may help to decrease potassium loss. Potassium rich foods include: bananas, oranges, tomatoes, and fish.
Loop Diuretics Furosemide* (Lasix®) Bumetanide (Bumex®) Torsemide (Demadex®)		Some people may have gout attacks since diuretics Can increase uric acid levels. May increase blood sugar in people with diabetes.	May have positive effect on cholesterol levels Make sure to wear sunscreen while exposed to the sun
Potassium Sparing Diuretics Spironolactone* (Aldactone®) triamterene plus hydrochlorothiazide* (Dyazide®,Maxzide®)		May cause sensitivity to the sun.	These agents will initially cause increased urination, you may want to take these pills in the morning to avoid getting up at night to urinate
Beta Blockers			
Acebutolol* (Sectral®), Atenolol* (Tenormin®), Metoprolol* (Lopressor®), Propranolol*(Inderal®) Timolol* (Blocadren®), Carteolol* (Cartrol®), Bisoprolol* (Zebeta®)	Decrease blood pressure by reducing the heart rate and output of blood from the heart.	Insomnia, cold hands and feet, tiredness or depression, slow heartbeat, worsen symptoms of asthma, impotence. May block the signs of low blood glucose such as increase heart rate. You should increase monitoring of glucose levels when starting these agents or when increasing the dose.	Drugs from this class are considered useful in patients that have a previous heart attack. Do not stop this medication suddenly without your provider's advice. This medication needs to be tapered down to the lowest effective dose.

*These drugs are available in generic, which means the generic alternatives are a cost savings to you!

Commonly Used High Blood Pressue Medications

ACE Inhibitors

Medications	Description	Notes
Captopril* (Capoten®), Enalapril* (Vasotec®), Lisinopril* (Zestril® or Prinivil®), Fosinopril (Monopril®), Quinapil* (Accupril®), Ramipril* (Altace®), Trandolapril* (Mavik®)	Interfere with the body's production of Angiotensin II. Angiotensin II is a chemical in the body that causes the arteries to constrict (tightening). By inhibiting this chemical, the ACE Inhibitors relax and dilate (widen) the blood vessels.	Many patients get a dry, hacking cough; if this continues consult with your provider. Can cause hives or swelling of the face or tongue Tell your provider right away if you experience any of these side effects Can increase potassium levels in patients with kidney dysfunction.	The best agents for patients with high blood pressure and diabetes. They protect the kidneys from damage. Do not use potassium supplements or salt substitutes containing potassium without consulting your provider.

Angiotensin II Receptor Blockers

Medications	Description	Notes
Candesartan (Atacand®), Irbesarten (Avapro®), Losarten (Cozaar®), Valsartan (Diovan®), Olmesartan (Benicar®), Eprosartan Teveten®), Azilsartan (Edarbi®)	Blocks the effects of Angiotensin II receptors. Decreases blood pressure by relaxing the blood vessels so there is less constriction (tightening)	Can increase potassium levels in patients with kidney problems	May be used in patients that experience a cough from ACE inhibitors. Do not use potassium supplements or salt substitutes containing potassium without consulting your provider These drugs protect the kidneys from being damaged.

*These drugs are available in generic, which means the generic alternatives are a cost savings to you!

Commonly Used High Blood Pressue Medications

NAME OF MEDICATION	HOW THEY WORK TO LOWER YOUR BLOOD PRESSURE	POSSIBLE SIDE EFFECTS	COMMENTS
	CALCIUM CHANNEL BLOCKERS		
Amlodipine* (Norvasc®), Felodipine (Plendil®), Diltiazem* (Cardizem®), Isradipine (DynaCircCR®), ® Nifedipine* (Procardia®, Adalat®), Verapamil* (Calan®)	Decreases blood pressure by relaxing the blood vessels of the heart	May cause increase in heart rate, swollen ankles, constipation, headache or dizziness	Notify your physician if you experience, shortness of breath, swelling of hands and feet, pronounced dizziness, constipation, nausea
	ALPHA BLOCKERS		
Doxazosin* (Cardura®), Prazosin* (Minipress®), Terazosin* (Hytrin®)	Decrease blood pressure by relaxing the blood vessels causing dilation (widening)	May cause increased heart rate, dizziness or a drop in blood pressure when you stand up	Upon starting dosage should be increased slowly. You should not stop taking this medication abruptly, it must be tapered. Better to take medicine at bedtime. Prescribed in men that have enlarged prostates
	CENTRAL AGONISTS		
Methyldopa* (Aldomet®), Clonidine* (Catapres®), Guanabenz (Wytensin®), Guanfacine (Tenex®)	Decrease blood pressure by inhibiting the nerve signals that come from the brain to the arteries of the body	Methyldopa may cause your urine to darken when exposed to air All can cause a fall in blood pressure when you stand up, weakness, fainting sensation, drowsiness, impotence, dry mouth, constipation and drowsiness	You should not stop taking these medications abruptly, taper down slowly You should use caution when starting these medications and when dose is increased may cause drowsiness/dizziness, do not drive or operate heavy machinery. Agents are better taken at bedtime

*These drugs are available in generic, which means the generic alternatives are a cost savings to you!

Commonly Used High Blood Pressue Medications

VASODILATORS

Vasodilators Nitrates- isosorbide dinitrate*(Isordil®), isorsobide mononitrate*(Imdur®), nitroglycerin sublingual* (Nitrostat®, NitroTab®, NitroQuick®) **Peripheral Vasodilators** Hydralazine (Apresoline®, Minoxidil®, Loniten®)	Decrease blood pressure by relaxing and dilating (opening up) the blood vessels	Nitrates may cause headaches, rapid heartbeat, light-headedness upon standing Peripheral Vasodilators may cause aches or pains in the joints	Do not use nitrates with erectile dysfunction agents Minoxidil is rarely used alone and is reserved for severe cases of high blood pressure. Can also promote hair growth

* These drugs are available in generic, which means the generic alternatives are a cost savings to you! † Swallow whole, co not crush or chew.

Figure 3: Heart Disease and Stroke Statistics 2007 update (Circulation. Rosamond et al 115(5):e69 2007)

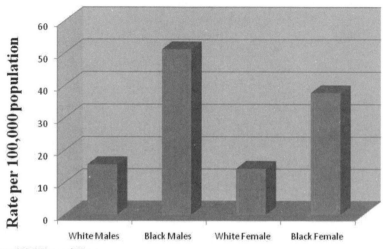

Test Your Knowledge
High Blood Pressure

1. High blood pressure causes

   a) blood vessels to get stiff and narrow
   b) weakening of the lining of the arteries and veins
   c) problems with the heart, kidney, brain and eyes

   1) a,b,d
   2) a,c
   3) b only
   4) all of the above

2. The proposed target blood pressure goal for African Americans is

   a) 150/90 mmHg
   b) 120/80 mmHg
   c) 140/90 mmHg
   d) 130/80 mmHg

3. African Americans have the highest rate of hypertension in the world

   TRUE   FALSE

4. The factors that contribute to high blood pressure in African Americans include:

   a) high salt diet
   b) sedentary lifestyle
   c) fewer physician visits
   d) genetic factors

   1) a,b,d   2) b,d   3) a,c   4) all of the above

Cholesterol and Heart Disease

What is Cholesterol?

Cholesterol is a soft, waxy substance found among the lipids (fats) in the bloodstream and in the body's cells. It is normal to have cholesterol. The body uses cholesterol for many functions, from building cells to making the bile acids that help digest fat. Cholesterol is an important part of a healthy body because it's used to form cell membranes, some hormones and other needed tissues. An elevated level of cholesterol in the blood is a major risk for coronary heart disease, which leads to heart attack. Hypercholesterolemia is the term used for high levels of blood cholesterol.

Two sources of cholesterol exist: the body makes some of it in the liver, while the rest is derived from animal products in the diet, such as meats, poultry, fish, eggs, butter, cheese and whole milk. It is made only in animals and in humans. Food from plants like fruits, vegetables and cereals do not have cholesterol. Saturated fat is a type of fat found in foods from animals. The greatest amounts of saturated fat are included in meat, dairy products, and some vegetable oils. These foods are high in cholesterol.

Triglycerides are another type of fat. As a major storage form of body fat it comes from two sources. It is produced by the body and is also ingested from dietary sources.

Cholesterol and other fats cannot dissolve in the blood and are carried to the tissues by special proteins called lipoproteins, which enable cholesterol to dissolve in the blood. **There are two major lipoprotein classes—high-density lipoprotein (HDL) and low-density lipoprotein (LDL).** It is important for you to know about lipoproteins since that is what your health care provider measures when they order a blood test for cholesterol.

LDL cholesterol (LDL-C) is the most important contributor to clogged arteries (known as atherosclerosis). A high level of LDL-C, often known as "bad" cholesterol, has been shown to increase the risk of heart disease.

HDL cholesterol, (HDL-C) or "good" cholesterol, contains mostly protein plus a small amount of cholesterol. HDL-C carries cholesterol away from the arteries and back to the liver, where it is passed from the body. High HDL-C levels are desirable, protecting against clogged arteries, while low HDL-C levels increase the risk of coronary heart disease. An easy way to remember the distinction between these two is that LDL-C is the "Lousy" or "Lethal" cholesterol, while HDL-C is the "Happy" or "Healthy" cholesterol.

Why do people with diabetes need to control their cholesterol?

It is very important that you control your cholesterol levels in the blood if you have diabetes. Over the years it has been proven that people with diabetes are more prone to getting heart disease and experiencing heart attacks and strokes. In fact, according to the latest guidelines of the National Cholesterol Education Program Adult Treatment Panel III (NCEP-ATP III) people with diabetes should consider their risk for heart disease the same as people without diabetes that have already had a heart attack. It appears that having abnormal blood fat (example: high triglycerides) in addition to high cholesterol levels contribute to increased heart disease risk. People with diabetes need to know their target level for blood cholesterol and take the necessary steps to lower their cholesterol levels to the normal range. A reminder of the seriousness of heart disease in diabetes is that heart attacks are the leading cause of death in people with diabetes.

How does lowering cholesterol lower heart attack risk?

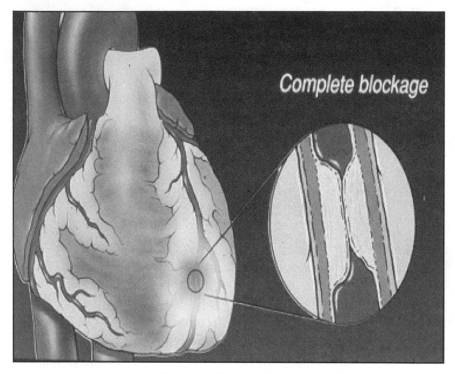

Complete blockage

Picture of Clogged Artery

The coronary arteries, located in the heart, are the "fuel sup-ply" to the heart muscle and provide blood for heart muscle contraction. Coronary artery disease is the process of cholesterol buildup within the walls of the coronary arteries. The heart attack occurs when a coronary artery becomes blocked and oxygen-rich blood can no longer get through to feed the heart muscle. The closure is caused by the buildup of cholesterol or more commonly when the cholesterol buildup (plaque) ruptures and a blood clot forms (Thrombus) and blocks the artery. This process of plaque rupture with clot formation is a more common occurrence in people with diabetes, contributing to heart attacks being the leading cause of death in diabetes.

What are the risk factors for coronary heart disease (CHD)?

The risk factors for CHD, as established by the National Cholesterol Education Program (NCEP-ATP III), include the following:

- Age (male > 45 years; female > 55 years or premature menopause without estrogen replacement therapy).
- Family history of premature CHD.
- Current cigarette smoking.
- Hypertension.
- Elevated total cholesterol.
- Low HDL cholesterol (< 40 mg/dL).

While certain risk factors (e.g., family history, age, gender) cannot be changed, others can be modified (changed). Modifiable risk factors for heart disease include smoking, hypertension, diabetes, and elevated blood cholesterol. In addition, patients can lose weight and increase physical activity to reduce risk.

Understanding High Cholesterol and Its Treatment

How many people in the United States have high cholesterol levels?

An estimated 105 million American adults have total cholesterol levels of 200 mg/dL and higher, while 42 million have total cholesterol levels of 240 mg/dL or greater.

For some people, a proper diet and physical activity can bring their cholesterol levels to the desired range to reduce their risk of heart attack and stroke. However, sometimes it may be necessary to take cholesterol-lowering medications in addition to diet and exercise to help achieve the desired range.

How often should you check your cholesterol levels?

It is generally recommended that all healthy adults over the age of 20 years have their fasting total cholesterol level measured at least once every 5 years. Fasting high-density lipoprotein cholesterol (HDL-C) should be measured at the same time if accurate results are available. Most patients with diabetes should receive a full lipid panel.

This panel includes the following measures:

- Total Cholesterol
- High Density Lipoprotein (HDL) Cholesterol
- Triglycerides

From these values the Low Density Lipoprotein (LDL) cholesterol is calculated. It is important to remember to not eat anything prior to getting your full lipid panel. Eating food 8-12 hour prior to the test will elevated you triglycerides and give you a falsely elevated LDL number.

When is the cholesterol level considered to be high?

The NCEP-ATP III guidelines include the following recommendations for initial classification based upon the following total cholesterol levels:

- Desirable: Less than 200 mg/dL
- Borderline-high: 200-239 mg/dL
- High: 240 mg/dL or above

In July 2004, the National Cholesterol Education Program (NCEP) redefined "high risk" and "very" high risk patients.

NCEP defines **high risk patients** as those with:

- Atherosclerotic heart disease

♦ Multiple risk factors (> 20% risk of heart attack in 10 years)

Very high-risk patients were those with:

♦ Cardiovascular disease plus multiple risk factors (especially diabetes)

♦ Severe and poorly controlled risk factors (e.g. smoking)

♦ Metabolic syndrome

♦ Hospitalization for acute coronary syndromes

For patient in these categories NCEP lowered the target LDL-C goal from 100mg/dL to 70mg/dL.

In order to achieve this lower LDL-C goal most patients will need to use more than one cholesterol lowering agent along with Therapeutic Lifestyle Change.

What are the nonmedical treatment options for high cholesterol?

Lifestyle changes

Diet, weight loss, and regular exercise are often the first steps prescribed to lower blood cholesterol and prevent heart disease.

Diets high in cholesterol and saturated fats can increase blood cholesterol levels. Foods from animal sources (meat, fish, poultry, dairy products) contain cholesterol. Organ meats, such as liver, are especially high in cholesterol. Although foods of plant origin have no cholesterol, they may contain types of dietary fats that increase blood cholesterol levels.

Reducing dietary fat and cholesterol can help people lose weight and lower heart disease risk factors. Limiting dietary cholesterol intake to 200 mg/day and eating a higher proportion of complex carbohydrates (bran, oatmeal and vegetable fiber) can lower cholesterol levels by an average of 10-15 percent and triglyceride levels by 15-20 percent.

What medications are used to control cholesterol levels?
HMG-CoA Reductase Inhibitors (Statins)

Statins have become the most frequently prescribed lipid-lowering drugs because they are highly effective in lowering LDL-C and are generally safe and well tolerated. Statins reduce cholesterol synthesis in the liver by inhibiting a key enzyme, HMG-CoA Reductase, which controls the cholesterol-producing process in the liver.

Clinical trials have demonstrated that statins significantly reduce LDL-C ("lethal" cholesterol), triglycerides, total cholesterol and minimally raise HDL-C ("healthy" cholesterol). In addition, long-term studies with some statins have demonstrated that LDL-C lowering through dietary modification and drug therapy reduces the risk of coronary heart disease illness and death. The statins are well tolerated with few side effects. If you are taking a statin, it is important that your health care provider periodically checks (2-3 times per year) your liver function.

Nicotinic acid

Nicotinic acid, or niacin, is a B vitamin that when used at lipid-lowering doses, can significantly reduce total cholesterol, LDL-C, and triglycerides. In addition, nicotinic acid raises HDL-C higher than any other lipid agent available today. Nicotinic acid can cause flushing and a headache. Some patients' find that taking an aspirin tablet 30 minutes before their niacin can help prevent or minimize flushing. Other recommendations to prevent flushing are avoiding spicy foods, hot beverages and alcohol around the time you take niacin, as well as, increasing the dose slowly over time. The longer you are on niacin, the less frequently flushing occurs. Nicotinic acid has the potential to raise blood sugar in persons with diabetes, with no or minimal change in Hemoglobin A1C, which is the determinant of your overall glucose control. Patients that have prediabetes and are at higher risk for developing diabetes and may have increased blood sugars on niacin, especially if they do not have a healthy lifestyle and are obese. However, the American Diabetes Association, American Association of Clinical Endocrinology, and American Heart Association recommend niacin as an alternative to improve the lipid panel because diabetics usually die of heart disease and not diabetes.

Bile acid-binding resins

The **bile acid-binding resins**, cholestyramine, colestipol and colesevelam, lower plasma cholesterol by binding bile acids in the intestine and inhibit their reuptake by the body. The subsequent increase in bile acid synthesis lowers the amount of cholesterol stored in the body. While less effective in reducing LDL-C levels, resins are often used in combination with statins for added LDL-C reduction. The bile acid resins can cause constipation so you should drink a lot of water. They also can interact with other medications (drug interactions) and therefore should be separated from your other medications by 1-2 hours.

Colesevelam (Welchol®)

Colesevelam a bile acid-binding resin used to lower cholesterol levels, has also been approved to help improve blood glucose control in adults with type 2 diabetes mellitus, in combination with other antidiabetic therapies such as metformin, sulfonyureas and insulin. To reduce the risk of complications associated with type 2 diabetes mellitus, there is need for simultaneous control of hyperglycemia, hypertension and dyslipidemias (increased lipids). Using Colesevelam in combination with other antidiabetic therapies may be of therapeutic benefit to you, by improving fasting glucose levels and decreasing A1C levels. The most common side effects associated with this drug were constipation and indigestion. This drug can interact with other medications and therefore should be separated from your other medications by about 1-2 hours. This drug is supplied in an oral powder form and as a tablet. The powder must be mixed with 4 to 8 ounces of water and should not be taken dry. The drug should be taken with a meal.

Fibric acid derivatives

The **fibric acid derivatives**, such as gemfibrozil and feno-fibrate, have a limited effect in lowering LDL-C and total cholesterol levels, but significantly lower triglycerides while raising HDL-C. These agents are well tolerated with few side effects.

Miscellaneous Cholesterol Lowering

Ezetimibe (Zetia®):

Ezetimibe is the first agent of the class of selective cholesterol absorption inhibitors. When given alone or in combination with a statin, fenofibrate, or niacin, ezetimibe reduces LDL-C by 15-20%, while increasing HDL-C by 2.5-5%. Ezetimibe does not adversely affect triglyceride levels. Patients who require modest LDL-C reductions or cannot tolerate other lipid-lowering agents are normally prescribed ezetimibe by itself. Patients who cannot tolerate high statin doses or in those who need additional LDL-C reductions despite maximum statin doses are normally prescribed ezetimibe with a statin.

Ezetimibe plus Simvastatin (Vytorin®)

Vytorin® is a combination of Ezetimide and Simvastatin, used to treat high cholesterol levels. Vytorin decreases total cholesterol and low-density lipoprotein (LDL) or "bad" cholesterol while increasing high-density lipoproteins (HDL) or "good" cholesterol. It is administered once daily in the evening with or with out food. The most common side effects of Vytorin® are headache, nausea, vomiting diarrhea and muscle pain. This drug should not be taken during pregnancy or by mothers who are breast-feeding their babies.

Omega-3- acid ethyl ethers (Omacor®)

Omacor® is a prescription omega-3 fatty acid formulation with high concentrations of eicosapentaenoic acid (EPA) (465 mg), docosahexaenoic acid DHA) (375 mg), and 4 mg (6 IU) of vitamin E. At a typical dose of 4 capsules/day, Omacor® significantly lowers plasma triglyceride levels by 45%. Omacor® also modestly increases plasma levels of LDL-C, minimally increases HDL-C levels. Omacor® may be used alone or in combination with statins, fibrates or niacin.

CLASS OF DRUG	HOW IT WORKS	WARNING	SIDE EFFECTS	COMMENTS
HMG-CoA Reductase Inhibitors				
Lovastatin* (Mevacor®, Altocor®, Altoprev®) Pravastatin* (Pravachol®) Simvastatin* (Zocor®) Fluvastatin* (Lescol®, Lescol XL®) Atorvastatin (Lipitor®) Rosuvastatin (Crestor®)	Reduces cholesterol synthesis by inhibiting the enzyme that makes cholesterol called HMG-CoA Reductase, in the liver.	Should be avoided in patients with -liver disease -pregnancy -breast feeding	May cause a rare side effect, muscle pain from myopathy (disease of the muscle)	All persons started on statins should be sure to report any muscle pain and weakness or brown urine
Bile Acid Binding Resins				
Cholestyramine* (Questran®) Colestipol (Colestid®) Colesevelam(WelChol®)	Bind to bile acids in the intestine and prevent them from being reabsorbed into the blood. The liver then produces more bile to replace the bile that has been lost. The body needs cholesterol to make bile; therefore the body uses up cholesterol in the blood thus lowering the LDL cholesterol circulating in the blood.	Should be avoided in patients with elevated triglyceride levels, > 400mg/dl	Bloating Fullness Constipation Nausea Gas	Bile Acid Binding Resins may interfere with the absorption of other drugs and vitamins. Colesevelam will not decrease the absorption of other drugs. Other drugs should be taken 1 hour before or 4 hours after taking these drugs. Cholestyramine and Colestipol are both administered as powders and should be mixed with water or juice.

*These drugs are available in generic, which means the generic alternatives are a cost savings to you!

Nicotinic Acid - Niacin

CLASS OF DRUG	HOW IT WORKS	WARNING	SIDE EFFECTS	COMMENTS
Time Release (Niacor®, Niacin - Time) **Extended Release** (Niaspan®) **Controlled Release** (Slo-niacin) *(These are the only nicotinic acid products available by prescription Other formulations are dietary supplements, purchased without a prescription Dietary Supplement niacin is not advised my most health organizations)*	- Reduces total cholesterol, LDL-C and triglycerides by preventing their formation - Increases HDL-C by preventing the breakdown, and increases the production of HDL-C	Should be avoided in patients with: - liver disease - severe gout - peptic ulcers	Flushing (More common with the immediate release forms) - Increased blood sugar - Increased uric acid - Stomach upset - Sustained release preparations have a tendency to cause problems with your liver, only available as a dietary supplement	To prevent flushing- Niacin should be taken during or after a meal, Take an aspirin 30 minutes before May want to avoid spicy foods, alcohol and hot beverages Slowly increasing the dose Niaspan® - is the only extended release, prescription once daily niacin formulation - has much less flushing than immediate release and - has less liver toxicity than sustained release

Fibric Acid Derivatives

CLASS OF DRUG	HOW IT WORKS	WARNING	SIDE EFFECTS	COMMENTS
Gemfibrozil* (Lopid®) Fenofibrate* (Tricor®, Lofibra® Tablets, Triglide®, Lipofen®)	Exact mechanism of action is unknown Fibrates are less effective in lowering LDL-C, but they improve HDL-C and triglyceride levels	Should be avoided in patients with: - liver disease - kidney disease	Mild Stomach upset Muscle Pain (Rare)	

CLASS OF DRUG	HOW IT WORKS	WARNING	SIDE EFFECTS	COMMENTS
Absorption Inhibitors				
Ezetimibe (Zetia®)	Prevents absorption of cholesterol	Should be avoided in patients with: - active liver disease - pregnancy - breast feeding	Stomach pain Tiredness Muscle Pain (rare)	Uexplained muscle pain or weakness could be a sign of a rare side effect, but should be reported to your health care provider
Omega-3-acid ethyl esters				
(**Omacor**®)	Exact mechanism of action is unknown. Omacor® reduces triglyceride levels	Should be used with caution in patients: - with known sensitivity or allergy to fish	Nausea Belching a fish taste Infection Flu symptoms Upset stomach Rash **Change in your taste buds**	Be careful taking this agent with other medications that thins the blood

*These drugs are available in generic, which means the generic alternatives are a cost savings to you!

Combination Cholesterol Drugs	Notes
Advicor® (Niacin + Lovastatin) Simcor® (Niacin + Simvastatin)	See Nicotinic Acids and HMG CoA Reductase Inhibitors
Caduet® (Atorvastatin + Amlodipine)	See HMG CoA Reductase Inhibitors and Calcium Channel Blockers Do not split or crush the tablets
Vytorin® (Simvastatin + Ezetimibe)	See HMG CoA Reductase Inhibitors and Selective Cholesterol Absorption Inhibitors

Test Your Knowledge
Cholesterol

1. Cholesterol is a soft, waxy substance found among the lipids (fats) in the bloodstream and in the body's cells. Increase levels of cholesterol can lead to coronary heart disease.

        TRUE   FALSE

2. Cholesterol comes from two sources.

    a)   Made in the Liver
    b)   Eating too many vegetables
    c)   Food that we eat
    d)   Eating high amount of monounsaturated fat

    1) a,b,c   2) b,d   3) a,c   4) all of the above

3. The name of the "Good" cholesterol that removes the "Bad" cholesterol from your body is called

    a)   LDL cholesterol
    b)   HDL cholesterol
    c)   Triglycerides
    d)   VLDL cholesterol

    1) a   2) b   3) c   4) d

4. People with diabetes need to control their cholesterol level in order to decrease their risk of heart attacks and strokes.

        TRUE   FALSE

Test Your Knowledge
Cholesterol

5. The risk factors for coronary heart disease are

    a) age, family history, hypertension, Low HDL cholesterol
    b) age, family history, low blood sugar, High HDL
    c) age, family history, low total cholesterol, low HDL cholesterol
    d) age, family history, low total cholesterol, current cigarette smoking

    1) a   2) b   3) c   4) d

6. Healthy adults over the age of 20 should check their cholesterol

    a) Every 2 years
    b) Every 5 years
    c) Every 10 years
    d) Every 15 years

    1) a   2) b   3) c   4) d

7. According to the NCEP-ATP III guidelines, a desirable total cholesterol value is

    a) Less than 300 mg/dL
    b) Less than 70 mg/dL
    c) Less than 200 mg/dL
    d) Less than 400 mg/dL

8. HMG-CoA Reductase inhibitors (Statins) have become the most frequently prescribed lipid-lowering drugs.
    TRUE   FALSE

Smoking Cessation

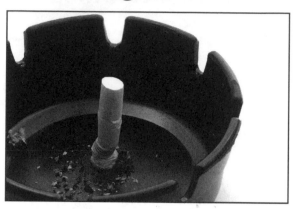

Why should I quit smoking?

One of the best things you can do for yourself and your loved ones is to quit smoking. Smoking is simply not good for you. This is especially true for people with diabetes. One out of every five deaths each year is caused by smoking. More than 443,000 died in 2007 in the United States from smoking. Smoking is considered to be the most preventable cause of illness and death in the United States.

Not only does smoking cause cancer and damages your lungs, it also is detrimental to your blood vessels and nerves throughout your body. Damage to the blood vessels in the heart, kidney, legs and feet causes hardening and narrowing of the vessels. In the heart and kidneys the destruction of these vessels accelerates both kidney and heart disease. In the lower extremities, foot and leg ulcers are slow to heal, due to the poor circulation. Infections can linger due to the negative impact of smoking, in which, poorly controlled glucose levels compound this problem. The narrowing of the blood vessels by smoking also increases blood pressure and worsens the cholesterol build up in your vessels. Smokers with diabetes are more likely to get nerve damage. People with diabetes cannot handle this extra stress on the heart. The chance of heart disease is much higher for smokers with diabetes than smokers without diabetes. Smoking has been shown to raise blood glucose levels, making diabetes harder to control.

Why is it so hard for me to quit?

Smoking is hard to quit for two reasons. One, tobacco contains nicotine, a very addictive substance. When you smoke, your body is tricked into thinking it needs nicotine every day. Therefore, when quitting, you may have symptoms of withdrawal. These symptoms include being irritable, sweating, headaches, hunger or being nervous. These symptoms will soon go away after a week or so.

Second, you may often think that you "need" to smoke. Smoking is part of what you do every day. If you are not smoking, you do not know what to do with your hands. As a smoker you may feel that a cigarette calms your nerves or gives you energy. These effects may last longer than the withdrawal symptoms, but they, too, will go away.

How do I quit smoking?

You must want to quit smoking. Your health care provider and your family and friends cannot quit smoking for you. You must be motivated to quit smoking and live a healthy life.

Now, more than ever, you have a number of ways to help you quit. You can simply quit smoking gradually by decreasing your use of tobacco on a daily or weekly basis or just quit altogether. Some experts regard quitting suddenly, also known as "cold turkey," as the most effective method of quitting smoking. This method of quitting smoking may be done with or without nicotine replacement products. You may want to talk to your health care provider about which plan will work best for you.

There are several products you can buy from your local pharmacy to help you quit smoking. These products contain nicotine in different strengths that will help wean you from smoking. You can try nicotine gums that you can chew and nicotine patches that you wear on your body. These nicotine products replace the nicotine found in tobacco. It is important for you to follow the directions that come with these products.

It is never too late to quit smoking. Once you quit smoking, it does not take very long for your lungs to heal themselves and for you to feel better. You will notice a positive change in your health and well being within weeks of quitting.

With the help of nicotine replacement products and encouragement from your friends and family, you could be on your way to a healthier smoke-free and happy life.

Table 19. Nicotine Replacement Products

NAME OF MEDICATION	DOSING	DURATION	SIDE EFFECTS
NICOTINE GUM - OTC* Nicorette 2 mg, 4 mg, Flavors: regular, mint (various), orange, cinnamon, fruit	> 25 cigarettes/day - 4 mg < 25 cigarettes/day- 2 mg Weeks 1-6: 1 piece every 1-2 hours Weeks 7-9: 1 pieces every 2-4 hours Weeks 10-12: 1 piece every 4-8 hours Maximum: 24 pieces/day	612 weeks	Unpleasant taste, mouth/jaw soreness, hiccups, upset stomach, nausea and vomiting, throat and mouth irritation. Do not chew gum too rapidly. Tell your doctor if you have stomach ulcers
NICOTINE LOZENGE - OTC Commit 2 mg and 4 mg Flavors: cappuccino, cherry, mint, original (light mint)	1st cigarette < 30 minutes after waking - 4 mg 1st cigarette > 30 minutes after waking - 2 mg Weeks 1-6: 1 lozenge every 12 hours Weeks 7-9: 1 lozenge every 2-4 hours Weeks 10-12: 1 lozenge every 4-8 hours Maximum: 20 lozenges/day	6-12 weeks	Nausea, hiccups, cough, heartburn, headaches insomnia, gas, mouth irritation. Tell your doctor if you have stomach ulcers Suck and rotate in mouth until the lozenge dissolves.
NICOTINE TRANSDERMAL PATCH - OTC Nicoderm CQ 7 mg, 14 mg, 21 mg 24 - hour release	>10 cigarettes/day 21mg/day X 6 weeks 14mg/day X 2 weeks 7mg/day X 2 weeks 10 cigarettes/day 14 mg /day x 6 weeks 7 mg/day x 2 weeks	8-10 weeks	Local skin reactions- redness, itching, burning, headache
Generic Patch (formerly Habitrol) 7 mg, 14 mg, 21 mg 24 - hour release	>10 cigarettes/day 21mg/day X 6 weeks 14mg/day X 2 weeks 7mg/day X 2 weeks 10 cigarettes/day 14 mg /day x 6 weeks 7 mg/day x 2 weeks	8 weeks	Local skin reactions - redness, itching, burning, headache, insomnia, vivid/abnormal dreams
NICOTINE NASAL SPRAY - RX Nicotrol NS Metered Spray 0.5mg nicotine in 50 uL aqueous nicotine solution	1 spray each nostril1-2 times/hour, at least 8 times/ day up to a MAX of 5 doses/hour; I dose = 2 sprays (one in each nostril) MAX: 40 doses/24 hours	3-6 months	Nasal and/or throat irritation, runny nose, tearing, sneezing, cough, headache

NICOTINE ORAL INHALER - RX Nicotrol Inhaler 10 mg cartridge delivers 4 mg inhaled nicotine vapor	Inhale with continuous puffing over 20 minutes: initial 6-16 cartridges per day up to 12 weeks. Gradually discontinue over 6-12 weeks. MAX: 16 cartridges/day; Nicotine is gone after 20 minutes of active puffing.	Up to 6 months	Mouth and/or throat irritation, unpleasant taste, cough, runny nose, upset stomach, hiccups, headache
BUPROPION SR - RX Zyban Sustained release tablet	150mg daily in the morning for 3 days, then increase to 150mg twice daily for 7-12 weeks. Do **NOT** exceed 300mg/day. Allow at least 8 hours between doses. Treatment should begin 1 week before the patient stops smoking. Set quit date for 1-2 weeks after stating therapy.	8-12 weeks	Insomnia, dry mouth, nervousness, rash, constipation, seizures
VARENICLINE TARTRATE Chanitx - RX	Days 1-3: 0.5 mg once daily Days 4-7: 0.5 mg twice daily Maintenance dose (day 8): 1 mg twice daily	12 weeks	Insomnia, headache, abnormal dreams, nausea.

OTC = Over the Counter   Rx = Prescription required

Test Your Knowledge
Smoking Cessation

1. More than 443,000 people died in 2007 in the United States from smoking.

   TRUE   FALSE

2. Smoking can cause the following problems

   a) Narrowing of the blood vessels
   b) Nerve damage
   c) High blood pressure
   d) Cancer

   1) a,b,c   2) b,d   3) a,c   4) all of the above

3. Some experts regard quitting suddenly, also known as "cold turkey," as the most effective method of quitting smoking.

   TRUE   FALSE

4. There are several smoking cessation products that you can buy at the pharmacy WITHOUT a prescription. The names of the products are:

   a) Nicorette™ gum
   b) Nicoderm CQ™
   c) Commit™ lozenge
   d) Zyban™ tablet

   1) a,b,c   2) b,d   3) a,c   4) none of the above

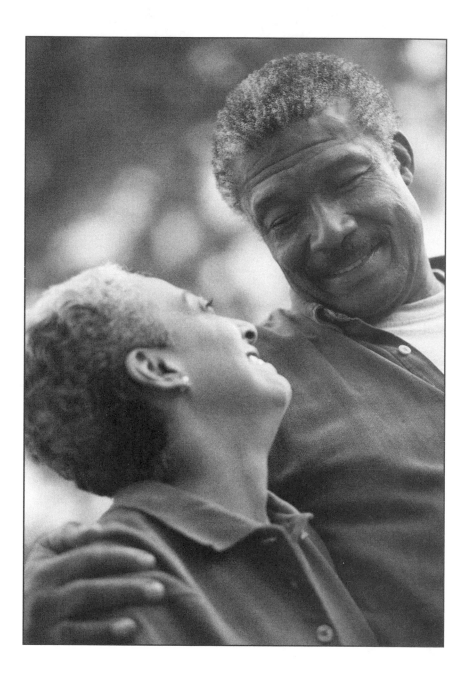

Section 5
Other Common Conditions

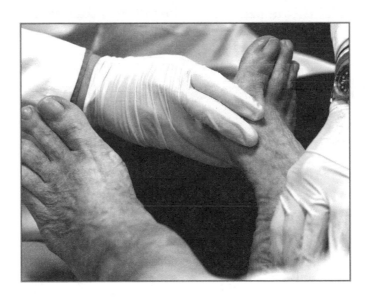

Types of Skin Conditions

Several kinds of bacterial skin infections occur in people with diabetes. Styes, carbuncles and infection of the nail beds may occur. Bacteria cause many infections. The most common bacteria is Staphylococcus also called Staph. If you think you have a bacterial infection, consult your health care provider.

Fungal infections are also seen in people with diabetes. Candida Albicans is a yeast-like fungus that causes the majority of the fungal infections. Common fungal infections include jock itch, athlete's foot, ringworm (a ring-shaped itchy patch), and vaginal infection. If you think you have a yeast or fungal infection, consult your health care provider. You may need a prescription medicine to cure it.

Acanthosis Nigricans is a skin disorder commonly seen in children with Type 2 diabetes. It appears as tan, brown or darkly pigmented raised areas that appear on the sides of the neck, armpits, and groin. Sometimes they also occur on the hands, elbows, and knees.

What should you do to take care of your skin?

Keeping your blood sugar levels as close to normal decreases your chances of getting a bacterial infection. Keep skin clean and dry, avoid very hot baths and showers and use talcum powder in areas where skin touches skin. To prevent dry skin it is important that you use moisturizing soaps and lotions on a daily basis. Lotions that are oil-in-water base are the best (Alpha Keri or Lubriderm). See a dermatologist (skin health care provider) about skin problems if you are not able to solve them yourself. Make sure you discuss your skin condition with your diabetes healthcare professional.

Taking Care of Your Feet

Why should I take care of my feet?

The longer you have diabetes, the more the blood glucose changes your body's blood vessels and nerves. The high blood glucose can actually damage the blood vessels and nerves so that they do not work as well. Over time, this can lead to foot problems.

Signs of possible foot/leg problems in people with diabetes:

- Sore on the foot or leg.
- Sore on foot or leg that does not heal.
- Infected sore (area around sore is red, raised or hot).
- Numbness or tingling (pins and needles sensation) in your feet.

The numbness and tingling are signs of nerve damage in your feet. Untreated foot problems can cause gangrene, a serious infection that can spread to the bloodstream. Untreated gangrene may lead to amputation of the foot.

With proper foot care and regular health care provider visits, you can avoid these foot sores or treat them before they become infected. It is important to see a foot health care provider (podiatrist) on a regular basis (at least 2 times per year).

1. Inspect your feet everyday for nicks, bruises, scrapes,

2. Make sure to check between your toes. If you have difficulty seeing the bottom of your feet, use a mirror. Also, check for changes in color or shape of your feet.

3. If you do develop a sore or blister, notify your health care provider immediately.

4. Wash your feet every day. When bathing, do not use very hot or very cold water. Test the water with your hand before stepping into the bathtub. Dry your feet carefully, especially between the toes.

5. Always wear socks or stockings with shoes.

6. Avoid high-heel and open-toed (such as sandals) shoes.

7. Wear only all-cotton (summer) or all-wool (winter) socks. Change your socks every day.

8. Do not use hot water bottles or heating pads on your feet. If your feet are cold at night, wear socks.

9. Never walk barefoot—even indoors.

10. Make sure that your shoes fit properly, not too tight or too loose. Shoes should be comfortable at the time of purchase. Do not depend on shoes to stretch out. It is best to have your feet fitted by a qualified shoe salesman who understands diabetes foot problems. Do not buy cheap shoes. Spending a little more money now may save you more money later by preventing sores on your feet.

11. Never wear new shoes more than 2 hours at a time. Inspect feet immediately after wearing new shoes for signs of redness, blisters, or swelling. Call your health care provider if these signs appear.

12. Inspect shoes on a regular basis for worn places, torn lining and rough areas. Do not put "over-the-counter" inserts into your shoes.

13. Change shoes twice a day, if possible.

14. Cut toenails straight across and gently round the corners with an emery board. If toenails are thick, have them trimmed by a podiatrist.

15. Never remove corns, ingrown toenails or calluses yourself. Have them removed by a foot health care provider (podiatrist).

16. Have your health care provider examine your feet on a regular basis. Take your shoes and socks off every time you see your health care provider to remind him/her to examine your feet.

17. Stop smoking.

18. Exercise on a regular basis. If your feet hurt during exercise, stop.

Dental Care

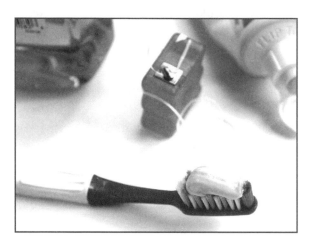

People with diabetes have an increased risk of gum disease and cavities. Diabetes may weaken your mouth's germ-fighting powers since it can affect your immune system. High blood sugar levels can cause or worsen gum disease.

Often gum disease is painless. You may not even know you have it until you have serious damage. Regular dentist visits are your best weapon. Some people with diabetes get oral infections (a cluster of germs) causing problems in one area of your mouth. Here are some warning signs: Swelling or pus around your teeth or gums, white or red patches on your gums, tongue, cheeks or the roof of your mouth, pain when chewing, dark spots or holes in your teeth. Fungal infections in the mouth may also occur if you blood sugar levels are high or you take antibiotics.

What can you do to prevent gum disease?

You should plan to see your dentist on a regular basis. Make sure they know you have diabetes. The best time for dental work is when your blood sugar level is in a normal range and your diabetes medication action is low. If you take insulin, schedule a morning visit after you eat a normal breakfast. Take your usual medicines before your dentist visit, unless your dentist or health care provider tells you to change your dose for dental surgery. Stick to your normal meal plan after dental work. If you can't chew well, plan how to get the calories you need. You may need to use your sick-day meal plan that uses more soft or liquid foods. Wait to have dental surgery until your blood sugar is in better control.

Erectile Dysfunction

The word "impotence" is used to describe emotional and physical conditions that may interfere with having sexual intercourse. People with impotence may lack the desire to have sex or have problems with orgasm or the release of semen (ejaculation of sperm during orgasm). Use of the words "erectile dysfunction" (ED) generally describes concerns with maintaining the erection of the penis. Erectile dysfunction may be experienced in varying degrees. You may have a total inability or inconsistent ability to achieve an erection and/or a tendency to sustain only brief erections. Many women experience sexual difficulties at some point in their lives as well.

Sexual Dysfunction in Men

Erectile dysfunction is commonly seen in men with diabetes. It occurs three times more often than in men without diabetes. Poor control of your blood sugar can lead to ED. Men with diabetes can experience the symptoms of ED in their 30s. A decrease in the quality of the sperm can lead to problems with infertility. You may also notice a lack of response to visual stimulation.

Sexual Dysfunction in Women

Sexual difficulties in women are usually seen during the late 40's. There are four categories of sexual dysfunction in women.

Desire Disorders – This is when you are not interested in having sex or has less desire for sex than you used to.

Arousal Disorders – Sometimes you may not feel a sexual response in your body or once aroused you are not able to maintain the arousal during sexual activity.

Orgasmic Disorders – When you can't have an orgasm even after sufficient sexual arousal and ongoing stimulation or you have pain during orgasm.

Sexual Pain Disorders – When you have pain during or after sexual stimulation or vaginal contact.

What are current treatment options for erectile dysfunction?

Psychotherapy and behavior modification in select patients are considered if indicated. Often psychologically based ED can be treated by using techniques that decrease anxiety associated with intercourse.

Fifty percent (50%) of the men with diabetes will have a psychological component to their ED. Decreased libido, fear of failure and diminished self-worth can be seen. Both controlling your blood sugar and talking with a counselor will be very helpful in dealing with the issues surroundings the management of erectile dysfunction.

Medication Therapy of ED

Medications utilized for treatment of ED can be taken orally, injected directly into the penis, or inserted in the urethra at the tip of the penis.

PDE Inhibitors: a class of drugs called phosphodiesterase (PDE) inhibitors. These drugs work by enhancing the effects of nitric oxide, a chemical that relaxes smooth muscles in the penis during sexual stimulation and allows increased blood flow into the penis resulting in erection.

Medications in this class include: Sildenafil (Viagra®), Vardenafil hydrochloride (Levitra®), Tadalafil (Cialis®). Men who take nitrate-based drugs such as nitroglycerin for heart problems should NOT use either oral or injected PDE drugs because the combination can cause a sudden drop in blood pressure. Oral testosterone can reduce ED in some men with low levels of natural testosterone; however, it is often ineffective and may cause liver damage.

Treatment of Sexual Dysfunction in Women

- Low sexual desire - Change your routine. Muscle relaxation exercises (contracting and relaxing your pelvic muscles) – "Kegel Exercises" (flexing the muscle that halts urination) can also help.
- Arousal disorders - can be helped if you use a vaginal cream for dryness.
- Orgasmic Disorder – Extra stimulation before sex can help.
- Pain during sex – try different positions. Using extra creams or try a warm bath before sexual intercourse.

Many men and women experience episodes of sexual dysfunction from time to time. If you take these steps, you can decrease the likelihood of occurrences. Limit or avoid the use of all forms of tobacco, avoid the use of alcohol, increase your activity, reduce your level of stress if it is interfering with your well-being and ability to function. See your health care provider for regular checkups and medical screening tests.

Depression

Depression results from abnormal functioning of the brain. Episodes of depression may then be triggered by stress, difficult life events, side effects of medications, or other environmental factors. Whatever its origin, depression can limit your energy so that it becomes difficult to focus on your treatment of other disorders, like diabetes. If you think you have depression you are not alone. In the U.S. it is estimated that 25 million people age 18 and older experience some form of depression. Depression is a serious medical condition that affects thoughts, feelings, and the ability to function in everyday life. Depression can occur at any age (7.4% of 9 to 17-year-olds have depression).

The rate of depression in people with diabetes is 3-4 times higher than people without diabetes. Studies have shown that 15-20% of people with diabetes also have depression. One large study actually showed that symptoms of depression can predict the incidence of Type 2 diabetes. People with diabetes may become depressed due to the stress of knowing they have a chronic disease that will change their daily routine. It is important that you recognize the signs of depression since depression can lead to an increase in diabetes complications. People that have both depression and diabetes have:

- Higher blood sugar levels and Hemoglobin A1C
- Decreased physical activity
- Higher rates of obesity
- More diabetic complications

Depression can lead to poor physical and mental functioning and/or not taking your medications as prescribed.

People with diabetes, their families and friends, and even their physicians may not recognize the symptoms of depression. However, skilled health professionals will recognize these symptoms and inquire about their duration and severity, diagnose the disorder, and suggest appropriate treatment.

What are the symptoms of depression?

Most people with depression will have several of the following symptoms listed below. These symptoms generally occur almost every day for at least a two (2) week period of time.

- Prolonged sadness or unexplained crying spells
- Significant changes in sleeping or eating patterns
- Irritability, anger, worry, agitation, anxiety
- Pessimism, indifference
- Loss of energy, lethargy
- Feelings of guilt, worthlessness
- Inability to concentrate, indecisiveness
- Inability to experience pleasure in former activities, social withdrawal
- Unexplained aches and pains
- Recurring thoughts of death or suicide.

Symptoms like these are normal after major losses, such as the death of a loved one, diagnosis of a new medical problem, or losing a job, but people should start feeling better after a few weeks.

Treatment for Depression

While there are many different treatments for depression, they must be carefully chosen by a trained professional based on the circumstances of the person and family. Prescription antidepressant medications are generally well tolerated and safe for people with diabetes. Antidepressant medications are widely used and effective treatments for depression. Antidepressant medications can take several weeks to work and may need to be combined with ongoing psychotherapy.

Specific types of psychotherapy, or "talk" therapy, also can relieve depression. It is important to see a professional—for example, a psychiatrist, psychologist, or clinical social worker.

Stress Management

Acute stress is the most common form of stress. It comes from demands and pressures of the recent past and anticipated demands and pressures of the near future.

Chronic stress destroys bodies, minds and lives. It wreaks havoc through long-term attrition. It's the stress of poverty, of dysfunctional families, of being trapped in an unhappy marriage or in a despised job or career. Chronic stress can be dangerous. It can cause suicide, violence, heart attack, stroke, and, perhaps, even cancer.

Stress can cause "wear and tear" on our bodies because of the continually changing environment. It has physical and emotional effects on us that can create positive or negative feelings. The personality of the individual and their environment can impact how stress is handled.

People with diabetes often find themselves feeling the symptoms of stress. Learning that you have a chronic disease and then finding out that you must make significant changes in your lifestyle can be very stressful.

Stress by itself can cause certain hormones in your body to be released. The "Stress Hormones" can actually cause your blood sugar to increase. Some people find that they feel less able to deal with stress when their blood glucose is out of control.

How does your body react to stress?

Your body secretes stress hormones (catecholamines, glucagon, cortisol and growth hormone) during times of stress. Symptoms that you may feel include nervousness, sweating, rapid heartbeat and nausea.

Tips for Managing Stress

Several activities to relieve stress:

- Take a deep breath and scan your body for physical tension
- Manage your time - do not overwork yourself and schedule too many tasks
- Get connected - join community groups, take a class, share your feelings with family and friend
- Make time for physical activity

Coping Skills

Listed below are a number of skills that can help you deal with the stress in your life.

- **Positive Coping Strategies** – tend to help you relax; Meditating, Exercise (Yoga), Interacting with friends and family
- **Negative Coping Strategies** – may make things worse such as, Drugs and Alcohol, Overeating, Sleeping all of the time.

Problem Solving

Every patient with diabetes has challenges and barriers to achieving and maintaining "good" control. Pick one problem at a time and begin the steps to solving that problem. If you follow these steps and asking yourself these questions you can begin the process of getting your blood sugar, blood pressure and cholesterol under better control.

Step 1 — Explore the Problem or Issue

- What is the hardest thing about caring for my diabetes
- Write down specific examples and review them with you educator

Step 2 — Clarify Feelings and Meaning

- Think about the problem that you are having and how it makes you feel

Step 3 — Develop a plan – Ask yourself the following questions

- What do you want to do?
- Where would you like to be with this problem 3 months from now?
- What are your options?
- What are your barriers?
- Who could help you?
- What would happen if you do nothing?
- How important is it, on a scale of 1 to 10, for you to do something?
- How confident, on a scale of 1 to 10, that you can make a change?

Step 4 — Commit to Action

- Are you willing to do what you need to do to solve this problem?
- What are some of the steps you could take?
- What are you going to do?
- When are you going to do it?
- How will you know if you are successful?
- What is the one thing you can commit to over the next 3 months.

Step 5 — Evaluate your success on a regular basis and reward yourself for the small steps. Modify your plan as necessary

HOW DOES YOUR BODY REACT TO STRESS?	STRESS
<ul><li>Stress hormones (catecholamines, glucagon, cortisol, and growth hormone)<ul><li>Symptoms (nervous, sweaty, palpitations, nausea</li></ul></li><li>How does stress effect diabetes and vice versa?</li><li>How does stress effect diabetes and vice versa?<ul><li>Increase blood glucose and ketones</li><li>Some people actually have a decrease in blood glucose initially</li></ul></li></ul>	<ul><li>What is stress?</li><li>Stress can be acute or chronic</li><li>Stress can occur when:<ul><li>An event produces a strain on a person</li><li>A person thinks a situation as challenging of threatening</li></ul></li><li>Stress is influenced by the<ul><li>Individual</li><li>Environment</li></ul></li></ul>

Test Your Knowledge
Other Conditions

1. Skin infections are very common in people with diabetes. The Candida Albicans is a yeast like fungus that causes the majority of fungal infections in diabetes.

   TRUE   FALSE

2. The signs of possible foot and leg problems in diabetes include:

   a) sore on foot or leg that does not heal
   b) itching
   c) numbness or tingling in your feet
   d) skin rash

   1) a,b,c
   2) a,c
   3) b,d
   4) all of the above

3. It is important to never walk barefoot, never soak your feet, and never wear shoes that are too tight or too loose.

   TRUE   FALSE

4. It is important to get dental checkups on a regular basis. The warning signs of a possible oral infection include:

   a) Swelling or pus around your teeth or gums
   b) White or red patches on your gums, tongue or roof of the mouth
   c) Pain when chewing
   d) Gaps between the teeth

   1) a,b,c   3) b,d
   2) a,c   4) all of the above

Test Your Knowledge
Other Conditions

5. Erectile Dysfunction (ED) is often seen in men with diabetes. The following statements are TRUE regarding ED.

    e) Men with diabetes can experience ED in their 30s.
    f) ED in diabetes is due to low blood sugar
    g) Men with ED may become infertile and lack a response to visual stimulation
    h) Women with diabetes DO NOT have problems with sexual dysfunction

    1) a,b,c
    2) a,c
    3) b,d
    4) all of the above

6. Depression results from abnormal functioning of the brain. People with diabetes have

    a) Depressions rate that is 3-4 times higher than people without diabetes
    b) Symptoms of depression that can actually predict the occurrence of Type 2 diabetes
    c) Symptoms of depression which include prolonged sadness, irritability, anger, worry, tiredness, feeling guilty and a inability to concentrate
    d) May need to see a psychiatrist or psychologist to teach them how to cope with their feelings regarding diabetes

    1) a,b,c
    2) a,c
    3) b,d
    4) all of the above

Section 6
Diabetes in the West Indies:
Focus on Myths and Misconceptions

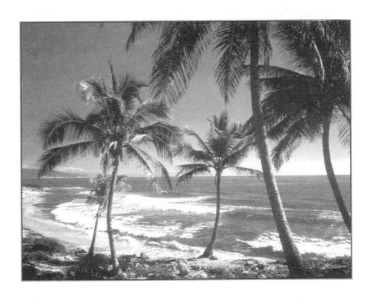

Introduction

The world-wide prevalence of Diabetes estimated by World Health Organization (WHO) was approximately 173 million in 2002 and is predicted to be at least 350 million by 2030. Approximately two-thirds of persons with diabetes live in developing countries. It has been estimated that one in six persons in Trinidad and Tobago has diabetes In 2000 was there were 60,000 people with diabetes and this number is projected to increase to 125,000 if the current trend prevails.

Though diabetes is a chronic and manageable disease the number of people dying from the complications of diabetes continues to increase. In 2005, an estimated 1.1 million people died from diabetes. We know that almost 80% of diabetes related deaths occur in poor countries. In Trinidad and Tobago diabetes death rates were the greatest (over 85 per 100,000). Approximately half of diabetes deaths occur in people under the age of 70 years with 55% of diabetes deaths occurring in women. The World Health Organization predicts that diabetes deaths will increase by more than 50% in the next 10 years.

Myths and Misconceptions

There are numerous myths and misconceptions that hamper the relationship between the person with diabetes and health care provider. These barriers are particularly relevant in the West Indies and also seen in ethnic minorities in the United States and United Kingdom. These barriers include socioeconomic problems, limited health literacy, language problems and cultural beliefs all of which impact on the provision of competent care. Tragically, these populations also have poor glucose control and are more likely to develop diabetes-related complications.

Some people with diabetes are in denial initially about their condition and seek religious or spiritual healing while refusing to visit the doctor. Occasionally, Hindus in Trinidad and Tobago and people from Guyana adopt a fatalistic view of their diabetes and believe that they are paying for their past sins ("karma"). Their diets are traditionally high in carbohydrates and fat with an increased risk of abdominal obesity.

Spouses are often fearful of "catching" diabetes from their partners and there is often marital discord when yeast infections are wrongly diagnosed as other sexually transmitted diseases. Additionally, the risk of being stigmatized as having erectile dysfunction makes many men in our "macho" societies deny that they have diabetes or even visit their doctor for this potentially treatable complication. It can also remain a dirty secret in persons who believe it is a "lazy man's disease" particularly as there may be few or no initial symptoms.

Diabetes Complications

In terms of diabetes complications lower extremity amputation rates in Barbados are among the highest in the world. The increase rates can be linked to inadequate footwear which actually tripled the amputation risk. Education of patients and healthcare professionals particularly about footwear and foot care is one key to reducing the risk of amputation.

Based on the information for the Barbados Eye Study we know that retinopathy was increased in patient with diabetes. The presence of retinopathy was much higher in type 1 patients (83%) versus type 2 patients (30%). Forty-one (41%) of patients in the study had cataract or a history of cataract surgery.

Heart disease, especially high blood pressure increases the risk of mortality in people with diabetes. The findings from Holder and Lewis indicated that mortality resulting from hypertension was highest in Dominica (over 90 per 100,000 of the population).

Diabetes in Children and Prediabetes

Despite the tsunami of diabetes amongst our children, many parents still believe that being overweight is a sign of good health.

Similarly, some women are afraid to lose weight as their husbands may no longer find them attractive. Obese persons with diabetes who lose weight are often ridiculed that they have contracted HIV/AIDS or cancer. The fact that there is still a social stigma attached to these conditions emphasizes the need for a widespread public health campaign. The fact that we are seeing more type 2 diabetes in children can be accounted for by (1) maternal nutrition during pregnancy, (2) diet and the environment. The sedentary lifestyles of the children and adolescents in the Caribbean population is further increased by the modern electronic games which have removed our young people from playing outside and competitive sports. We now see our children spending longer periods of time on the couch in front of the television or on the internet. This "hooked-on-technology" phenomenon has resulted in the increased consumption of fast foods, sweet snacks and junk food.

Prediabetes

There has been renewed interest in the burgeoning incidence of "prediabetes" or persons "at risk for diabetes". Many studies have shown the value of lifestyle changes or certain medications in delaying the progression to diabetes in such individuals. Yet, many patients are told that they have a "touch" or "trace of sugar" without adequate follow-up, monitoring or treatment. Indeed, many are surprised to learn when they present to hospitals with problems affecting their eyes, kidneys, nerves, feet and heart that they have had undiagnosed diabetes for decades. In the vain hope that they will be told that they no longer have diabetes, some persons begin "doctor-shopping" upon diagnosis which often worsens their control.

Diabetes and Nutrition

Many persons with diabetes are not referred for appropriate nutritional counseling and wrongly believe that they cannot eat anything sweet and "too much sugar" caused their diabetes. Thus, some embark on "starvation" diets and may become depressed due to the severe calorie restriction. Not eating regular meals can cause frequent low sugar levels ("hypoglycemia" = "hypos") requiring treatment.

The popularity of "bush" teas made from periwinkle, rice bitters, carailli (Momordica charantia), aloe vera and olive bush (Bontia daphnoides) have been used by persons with diabetes in the Caribbean especially those with numbness or tingling in the feet, weakness and dizziness. Some rural communities in Trinidad and Tobago also believe that eating wasps' nests will lower blood sugar. Many patients still insist that "white rum" is enough to control their diabetes despite the fact that it is a byproduct of sugar-cane and may cause "hypos" particularly in those with a background of poor nutrition. Unfortunately, some of these home remedies not only interfere with medications prescribed by physicians but have not been scientifically tested and are often used in preference to proven therapies. In the West Indies and throughout the Caribbean people with diabetes seek out modern "snake-oil" vendors claiming they have a "cure" for diabetes. It imperative that you are aware of the potential risks of these unproven therapies and have frank discussions with your doctor and healthcare team.

Information on Medication Use in the West Indies

Apart from the fear of injections, insulin is unfortunately associated with anxiety amongst both patients and health care providers. There is a common misconception that insulin means you have a "bad" type of diabetes and death is near. Many West Indian patients particularly Hispanics and those of African descent believe that insulin can cause complications like blindness and kidney disease. The truth is insulin therapy is often initiated too late in the disease. When initially diagnosed with diabetes, you should remember that insulin is not a threat but can greatly improved your diabetes control and decrease and/or slow the progression of many long term complications. Insulin is a hormone that plays a role in a human being's normal sugar control and is being replaced when necessary to prevent complications. Many patients do not want to start insulin due to the fear of needles. The fear of needles may have originated from the antiquated vaccination equipment that could have terrorized patients early in their childhood. Starting on insulin does not necessarily mean that you have failed in your diabetes management but represents a wonderful way for you to achieve near normal blood glucose levels.

Use of Technology and New Devices

Over the last 10 years there has been a great deal of improvements in insulin injection and blood glucose monitoring devices. The use of insulin pens may not be as forbidding as the traditional vial and syringe. It is our experience that using insulin pens can greatly improve insulin taking behavior and improve adherence.

Interestingly, a study in April 2011 in the United States showed that the use of glucose monitors and at-home record-keeping improved outcomes for poorly-controlled Type 2 diabetes - by prompting their doctors to put them on insulin faster. The apparent reluctance or "inertia" to commence insulin is thus reduced. Some people with diabetes are unable to afford or are afraid of fingerprick blood testing and believe that the absence of sugar in their urine implies good glucose control. You should remember that the blood glucose level must be monitored as it may be high with no spillage into your urine.

Low Blood Sugar (Hypoglycemia) Reactions in People with Diabetes

It is important that you are aware of the signs, symptoms and treatment of hypoglycemia. In my practice I have been told by patients that indeed, some Type 1 diabetes patients are thought to be demon-possessed during low blood sugar (hypoglycemia) episodes – with possible deadly consequences. As many as two-thirds (2/3) of people with type 1 diabetes may experience nighttime hypoglycemia.

In summary, we know that providing culturally competent care, healthcare providers must be sympathetic and understanding. It is critical that you communicate with your physician and learn as much as possible. There must be mutual respect and ongoing communication between you and your doctor so that you become empowered to take control of your condition. Healthcare providers and patients must work together to overcome the myths, misconceptions, psychosocial, cultural and ethnic barriers in order to provide excellent care and ultimately **"Heal Our Village."**

Test Your Knowledge

Diabetes in the West Indies

1. Obesity and Type 2 diabetes are becoming more common among children.

    TRUE   FALSE

2. Insulin is only started when a person with diabetes is going to die soon.

    TRUE   FALSE

3. Your neighbor recommends a new "natural" herbal remedy to control blood sugar. What should you do?

    a) Start using it at once and stop your other medications
    b) Use half the dose
    c) Try it out on your mother-in-law first
    d) Talk to your doctor about any medications before use

    1) a,b,c
    2) a,c
    3) b,d
    4) d only
    5) all of the above

Section 7
General Diabetes
Information and Resources

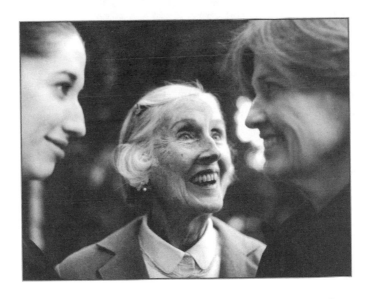

Goal Setting

Living every day with diabetes can have an impact on all aspects of your life. Many patients find it overwhelming and just give up. One way to manage your diabetes more effectively and to decrease your stress is to set reachable goals. Setting goals will keep you on track and also help you see that you are making progress.

What are the steps for setting goals?

Step 1 — Identify the changes you want to make

Step 2 — Identify the steps you need to take to make the changes

Step 3 — Break the changes down into the following categories

Small

Achievable

Challenging – not too easy

Step 4 — In order for change to be made a permanent part of your life you must change your behavior. The behavior changes needs to be something that you WANT to do and CAN do.

Step 5 — Develop a plan for carrying out the change

- What am I going to do?
- How much am I going to do?
- When am I going to do it?
- How often am I going to do it?
- How confident am I that I will achieve this goal?

Areas of your life where you can set goals?

Healthy Eating – Examples include: Reducing your fat; reducing portion sizes of your meals, using a smaller dinner plate or increasing your vegetable and fruit intake by eating fruit at each meal or for your snacks

Physical Activity – Examples include: Starting an exercise program with a friend or your family. Make it fun; dancing, bicycling, water aerobics, tennis, etc; increasing your activity level at your workplace

Monitoring – Increasing the number of times per week or per day that you test your blood sugar; keeping a log book or using a computer based tracking software. Reviewing your blood sugar levels before and after meals, exercise or after taking your medication

Medications – Taking your prescribed medication at the correct dose and time every day; site rotation if taking insulin or keeping a record of the medications you take

Reducing risk – Following the 'Rule of 15' for all blood sugars less than 70mg/dL or checking ketone level if you have Type 1 diabetes or if you are sick

Keeping well – Keeping health care visits with you doctor; going to a diabetes education class or support group at least at once per year, checking your feet daily and having your eyes checked at each visit

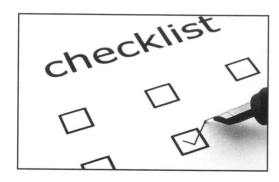

Checklist for General Good Health

If you have diabetes there are certain things that you must do on a regular basis. Think of it as your "bill of rights." You must work with your health care provider to make sure that you have all of the blood tests and examinations that are recommended to keep your diabetes under control and be monitored for short and long-term complications.

Foot care

- ◆ Check your feet everyday.
- ◆ Wash your feet everyday.
- ◆ Keep your toenails cut and clean.
- ◆ Keep your feet protected.
- ◆ Exercise everyday to improve circulation.
- ◆ Have your health care provider check your feet at every visit.

Eye care

- ◆ Have your eyes checked by an eye specialist (ophthalmologist) every year.
- ◆ If you have blurred vision, see dark spots, or have pressure or pain in your eyes you need to be seen as soon as possible.
- ◆ Check your blood pressure often but definitely at every health care provider visit. Make sure your health care provider

shares your blood pressure reading with you at every time it is measure. Goal for blood pressure in people with diabetes is less than 130/80 mmHg.

Skin care

- Take a bath everyday.
- Protect your skin to avoid cuts and scrapes.
- Treat any cuts or sores right away.
- Show your health care provider any cuts or sores that do not heal.

Dental care

- Use good dental hygiene (brush and floss everyday).
- Visit your dentist every 6 months.
- Make sure your dentist knows you have diabetes.

Guidelines for Monitoring Diabetes Control

EXAMS	RECOMMENDED STANDARDS	FREQUENCY
Hemoglobin A1C value (%)	Less than 7%	2-4 times a year (unless you are at your target value)
Blood Sugar (Capillary Plasma Glucose) Using Blood Glucose Monitor at Home	90-130 mg/dL	Type 1 diabetes—3-4 times/ day Type 2 diabetes 1 - 2 times/ day
Blood Pressure	Less than 130/80 mmHg	Every Visit
Foot Exam	Done by Primary Care Provider	Every Visit
Eye Exam	Done by Eye Specialist	Yearly
Urine Protein	Less 30 ug/mg	Every Visit
Body Weight (BMI)	25 kg/m2	Every Visit
Lipids Low Density Lipoprotein Cholesterol (LDL-C, Bad Cholesterol)	Less than 70 mg/dL	Yearly (Note: Should be done more frequently if not controlled)
High Density Lipoprotein Cholesterol (HDL-C, Good Cholesterol)	Greater than 40 mg/dL in men Greater than 50 mg/dl in women	At least yearly and more often if needed to achieve goals
Triglycerides	Less than 150 mg/dL	At least yearly and more often if needed to achieve goals.
Cholesterol	Less than 200 mg/dL	At least yearly and more often if needed to achieve goals
Nutrition Counseling	Individualized Medical Nutrition Therapy by Registered Dietitian	Recommended for all patients on a regular basis

Resources for More Diabetes Information

How can I learn more about my diabetes?

Education is the keyword. Read everything you can about diabetes and how you can control it. You should use this information along with any help given to you by your health care provider, nurse, dietitian, pharmacist or other diabetes educators. There are many groups in the United States that can provide valuable information to diabetic patients and their families.

The U.S. government has made an abundance of useful material about diabetes prevention and management available through the National Diabetes Education Program (NDEP). The American Diabetes Association (ADA) is an excellent provider of diabetes material. They can provide you with anything from diabetic cookbooks to information on the best blood glucose monitor to purchase.

American Diabetes Association
1701 North Beauregard Street
Alexandria, Virginia 22311
800 342 –2383
www.diabetes.org

American Association of
Diabetes Educators
100 W. Monroe #400
Chicago, Illinois 60603
800 338-3633
www.aadenet.org

National Institutes of Health,
National Institute of Diabetes
& Digestive & Kidney Diseases
Building 31, Room 9A04
31 Center Drive
Bethesda, Maryland
20892-2560
www.niddk.nih.gov

National Diabetes Information
Clearinghouse
1 Information Way
Bethesda Maryland
20892-3560
301 654-3327
800 860-8747

American Dietetic
Association
120 South Riverside Plaza
#2000
Chicago, Illinois 60606-6995
800 877-1600
www.eatright.org

National Diabetes Education
Program
800 438-5383
www.ndep.nih.org

National Eye Institute
National Institutes of Health
2020 Visions Place
Bethesda Maryland
20892-3665
301 496-5248
www.nei.nih.gov

National Center for Chronic
Disease and Prevention and
Health Promotion (CDC)
1600 Clifton Road
The Rodes Building, MS
K-13
Atlanta, Georgia 30333
404 639-3311 / 800-311-3435
www.cdc.gov/netinfo.htm

Conclusion

Diabetes is a common chronic disease that occurs more frequently in people of color. It is important to get an early diagnosis and start treatment as early as possible. Tight control of your blood sugar will help to delay and/or prevent the long-term complications of diabetes. People with diabetes have increased risk of blindness, kidney disease, heart disease, and amputation. All of these complications improve with better control of your diabetes.

Your goal for your blood sugar is a before meal sugar (fasting) between 90-130mg/dL, two hours after meal (postprandial) sugar less than 180 mg/dL and your Hemoglobin A1C below 7%. Eating a low fat, low carbohydrate diet, exercising 4-5 times per week for 30 minutes and taking your medications as prescribed can achieve your blood sugar goals. If you are not at your A1C goal and have been on oral diabetes medications for some time, ask your health care provider about insulin. Often, one to two shots a day of insulin with your oral medications can help you achieve your A1C goal. Since diabetes is a progressive disease it is possible that you will eventually require multiple insulin injections. The good news is that insulin therapy is much better today than it was 10 years ago. We now have new insulin products that mimic the body's natural secretion of insulin. These newer insulins cause fewer side effects and are well tolerated by most patients without problems.

Only you can make difference in your diabetes control. Though your health care provider can advise you and prescribe medications for you, it is your responsibility to keep track of your progress. Make sure that during your every 3-month health care provider visit you have your FEET CHECKED. Remember to WRITE down your:

- BLOOD PRESSURE READING
- CHOLESTEROL VALUES
- A1C VALUE

DISCUSS THESE VALUES WITH YOUR HEALTH CARE PROVIDER! ASK THEM IF YOU NEED TO CHANGE YOUR MEDICATION THERAPY.

Every year you need to have

- Your Eyes Checked
- Complete physical exam
- See your Podiatrist and Dentist

We recommended that every person with diabetes be seen by a **Registered Dietitian** to discuss meal planning and calorie control. A dietitian will help you learn to plan your meals and suggest low-fat cooking techniques to help you achieve and maintain your ideal body weight.

If you have Type 2 diabetes, make sure that everyone in your family that are undiagnosed are screened for diabetes. Screening is recommended every 3 years beginning at age 45 in people who are overweight (BMI > 25 kg/m²) with a family history of diabetes. If your are African American, Latino, Native American, Asian of Pacific Islander screening should be done at 35 years of age.

Controlling your diabetes is possible and will help you to live a longer, healthier life. Monitoring your blood sugar at home and writing down your numbers is the first step to better diabetes control. Remember, no one can take care of you and cares more about you than YOU. You are your "PRIMARY CARE PROVIDER." Only YOU can make a difference in your life with diabetes.

Test Answer Key

About Diabetes
1) d   2) all of the above   3) b,d   4) a,b,c

Risk Factors
1) All of the above   2) b,d

Hyperglycemia
1) a,b,c   2) a,b,c   3) TRUE

Hypoglycemia
1) FALSE   2) All of the above   3) TRUE   4) a,b,d   5) TRUE

Monitoring Blood Glucose
1) TRUE   2) a,b,c   3) c   4) All of the above

Diabetes and Nutrition
1) TRUE   2) TRUE   3) All of the above   4) TRUE   5) TRUE

6) a,c   7) d only

Obesity and Exercise
1) d   2) TRUE   3) All of the above   4) All of the above

5) b   6) TRUE

Oral Antidiabetic Medications
1) TRUE   2) All of the above   3) b,d

Test Answer Key

Injectable Antidiabetic Medications

1) All of the above   2) FALSE   3) All of the above   4) TRUE

Health Literacy

1) TRUE   2) a,c   3) TRUE   4) TRUE   5) a

Diabetes Complications

1) a,b,c   2) TRUE   3) a,b,c   4) TRUE

High Blood Pressure

1) All of the above   2) b   3) TRUE   4) All of the above

Cholesterol

1) TRUE   2) a,c   3) b   4) TRUE

5) a   6) b   7) c   8) TRUE

Smoking Cessation

1) TRUE   2) All of the above   3) TRUE   4) a,b,c

Other Conditions

1) TRUE   2) All of the above   3) TRUE   4) a,b,c

5) a,c   6) All of the above

Diabetes in the West Indies

1) TRUE   2) FALSE   3) d only

BOOK ORDER FORM

BOOK AVAILABLE THROUGH

Healing Our Village Publishing

www.healingourvillage.com

Healing Our Village: *A Self-Care Guide to Diabetes Control*   **$14.95**

Healing Our Village Publishing
10104 Senate Drive #201
Lanham, MD 20706
(800) 788-0941
(301) 577-1655 FAX

Name_____ Date_____

Address_____

City_____ State____ Zip Code_____

Day Telephone_____

Evening Telephone_____

Book Title_____

Number of books ordered_____ Total...... $ _____

Sales Taxes................................ $ _____

Shipping & Handling $3.90 for one book ..... $ _____

Add $.30 for each additional book .... $ _____

Total Amount Due........................ $ _____

__ Check   __ Money Order __ Other Cards_____

__ Visa   __ MasterCard Expiration Date_____

Credit Card No._____

Driver License No._____

Make check payable to: Healing Our Village Publishing

_____

Signature   Date